Have you tried to lose weight,
but found it impossible to stick with
a diet plan?

Have you lost weight, but see the
pounds creep back?

Have you been heavy for so long that
you think it can never change?

Have you almost given up hope?
HELP IS HERE.

You *can* be thin—for the
rest of your life!

Find out how, in . . .

Thin Tastes Better

THE "DIET BOOK" THAT TELLS YOU WHAT OTHER BOOKS CAN'T . . . OR WON'T.

- Ground rules for living in a house full of food

- The ten commandments of going food shopping

- Times of the day and week when you are most likely to meet a food trigger

- How to handle a dietary slip

- Discover your Eating Print—your unique history with food

- Eliminate the craving for "treats" and "goodies" that make you lose control

- Self-talk that works a diet miracle and even . . .

- Excellent weight loss centers if you need a jump start on your way to thin

**"The only new thing to come along in the field of weight control since the word 'diet' was invented."
—Dr. Austin Kutscher, Administrative Chair, National Obesity and Weight Control Education Institute, Columbia-Presbyterian Medical Center**

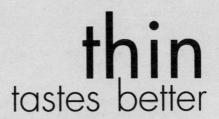

thin
tastes better

Control Your Food Triggers
and Lose Weight
Without Feeling Deprived

STEPHEN P. GULLO, Ph.D.

FOREWORD BY ARTEMIS P. SIMOPOULOS, M.D.

A Dell Book

Published by
Dell Publishing
a division of
Bantam Doubleday Dell Publishing Group, Inc.
1540 Broadway
New York, New York 10036

The information and guidelines in this book are not intended to replace professional medical advice. Before starting this or any other weight-loss program, consult with your physician, and continue to be monitored by your physician while you are losing weight.

The case histories recounted in this book are all based on actual clients. However, to protect their privacy, names and some distinguishing characteristics have been changed.

ISBN: 0-440-22231-1

Reprinted by arrangement with Carol Southern Books

Printed in the United States of America

Published simultaneously in Canada

March 1996

10 9 8 7 6

OPM

To my late mother, Rose Pernice Gullo, whose
unconditional love and caring was the source of my
inspiration to help others

To Joseph Amodio and Catherine Heusel, whose
gifted intellects and pens helped to make this
book a reality

To the women and men, my clients, whose
continued strivings and successes in self-mastery
with food are the source of my strength and renewal

ACKNOWLEDGMENTS

Many people have nurtured both my life and work and I will always be grateful to them. Truly, if I had every success in my profession and every material comfort and I did not have these deep abiding relationships, my life would be incomplete.

My family has loved and supported me unconditionally, and to my sisters, Angela Barna, Marianne Froelich, and Antoinette Pahlck; my nephews and niece, Christian Hanny, Matthew Touron, and Maurene Levine; and my brothers-in-law, Joseph Barna, Allan Froelich, and Robert Pahlck, I say *thank you*. I have also been blessed with a loving second family in a special woman, Choi Ping Roland, and Mathew and Lee Love, along with Florence Lazar, Al Galleau and Wendy, Kurt and Lance Barnard. You have all been and always will be a source of inspiration for me.

Along the road of my life many friends have made enormous contributions to my growth: David and Marilyn Kohn, Drs. Daniel and Justine Carr, Michael and Marjorie Francis, Jason Capuano, Dr. Dan Cherico, Dr. Marc Shatz, Dr. Henry Berger, Will Geurts, Peter Swersey, John Contini, Lenin De La Cruz, Gloria and Louis Flanzer, Steve Zubkoff, Fran Brody, Andrew Lassman, Ronni Janoff-Weinstein, Scott Yacker, Bernadette Baer, Diane Handler, Madeline Batagliese, Dee Kerner, Jaron Eames, Paul Ortiz, Mike Nelligan, Janet Goldman, Carol Ginsburg, and, of course, my dear friends and associates Edoardo Danilan,

Rosemarie and Tom Passaro, and Norbert Bogner. I am particularly grateful for the personal and professional support given to me and my work by my esteemed friends Jack Rudin and Nuno and Muriel Brandolini.

Michael Swiander, my research associate and colleague, did so much of the painstaking and outstanding work that helped me formulate my theories of Food Control Training.

At critical points in my development, I was able to call on the wisdom of several professors who enhanced my life with their guidance: the late Dr. Boyd McCandless, Dr. Rosalea Schonbar, Dr. David Peretz, the late Dr. B. Schoenberg, Dr. Ivan Goldberg, and, most of all, Dr. Austin Kutscher—all brilliant educators who inspired my career and my life. I am also grateful for the counsel and wisdom shared with me by the Rev. Harold Robertson, Dr. R. Corriere, and Dr. L. Hatterer.

I want to express special words of appreciation to Cindy and Gary Wattenberg, who have introduced me to many products and nutritional supplements that are helping a large number of people.

Each week I call on the professional expertise of a group of gifted advisors: Dr. David Kohn, Michael Kalnick, and Marvin Weinstein. Their guidance has enabled me to navigate around so many of life's pitfalls.

Susan Knightly provided invaluable assistance with recipes and cooking skills, and Dr. Shari Lieberman, distinguished nutritionist, served as nutritional consultant, sharing many important insights. I am grateful to these two leading professionals for their caring and assistance.

In recent years a number of outstanding people have entered my life and shared their friendship and expertise with me. Their insights have left an indelible mark on my professional and personal growth. No words can ever express the gratitude I feel to my dear friend Alexandra Penney, whose rare generosity of spirit and professional brilliance have so meaningfully shaped the present and future course of my career. Ruth Edelman has been one of the world's best teachers and loyal friends. Her words guide me in so many of the steps I will take into the future. Daniel and Rene Edelman have also been very generous with their time and expertise, and I have great appreciation for all that I have learned from them. Nancy Novogrod was the first person to encourage me to bring this book to Crown/Carol Southern Books; her wisdom helped me at a most critical time and I will always be appreciative of this support.

In the writing and marketing plan for this book so many individuals shared generously with me their invaluable guidance. Carol Southern has been a most gifted editor, counselor, and friend. This book would never have become a reality without her vision and support. My respect for this singular human being is boundless. I have also found in the executive and professional staffs of Crown/Carol Southern Books gifted leaders and individuals who supported and shaped this book: Michelle Sidrane, president of Crown Publishers, Barbara Marks, Robin Strashun, Eliza Scott, Camille Smith, Laurie Stark, and Joy Sikorski, all of whom have been enormously helpful.

Robert Barnett, Esq., of Williams & Connolly, was the erudite and gifted attorney who made possible the sale of this book and who once again proved the wisdom of our mutual friends, Ruth and Daniel Edelman.

Richard Rubinstein and Carolyn Carter helped enormously in selecting the title for this book and in graciously teaching me so many of the fundamentals of marketing. I also thank Melanie Radley for her guidance and insight during the years of our friendship.

Bob Bender was my first editor in writing a book for the lay public. He encouraged my writing and I will always feel a bond of great esteem for his talents and humanity. Catherine Heusel and Joseph Amodio were the most talented writers who shaped this book and made it possible. *Thin Tastes Better* is a tribute to their writing skills.

Several of my talented clients and friends were generous enough to share their personal recipes with me. I thank each one of you not only for myself but for the many readers who will benefit.

No set of acknowledgments for this book could fail to mention the role of a group of people I admire and esteem greatly: my clients. We have learned a great deal from each other, and their experience and successes form the basis for Food Control Training. In a very real sense they have been my coauthors, and I am most grateful.

Lastly, I have only one regret—that my late mother, Rose Pernice Gullo, is not here to see this book. Through her love and caring she has shaped all that I have done and will do in my life. My gratitude and respect for this woman I was blessed to call "mother" is eternal.

CONTENTS

MENUS, RECIPES, AND RESOURCES

FOREWORD

By Artemis P. Simopoulos, M.D.
President, The Center for Genetics, Nutrition and Health

Obesity is the most common nutritional disorder of Western culture and is becoming one in the developing world as well. For years we have known that obesity runs in families, and recent studies suggest that genes are involved. But just because one is predisposed to obesity, one does not have to become obese.

The majority of us are not obese, as we are able to maintain a balance by watching what we eat in relation to how much energy we expend. In other words, we have been able to *control* our weight. About one third of us are obese because either we eat too much or we are too sedentary, or both, causing an imbalance between energy intake and energy expenditure.

Hippocrates was the first person to recognize the morbid aspects of obesity. "Death comes early in the obese," he stated, and admonished the people and the physicians of his time to move and exercise.

Why is 30 percent of the U.S. population in this condition? One reason is that muscular work, which accounted for 30 percent of energy expenditures at the turn of the century, only accounts for 1 percent today, since the advent of machines. In the United States, Canada, and Britain, the three Western cultures with the largest number of obese people, sedentary lifestyles, lack of exercise, and a very palatable food supply based mostly on easily obtainable processed food, appear to be the leading causes of obesity.

This obvious market of obese people has led to commercial weight loss and exercise programs, which have been able to help people lose weight successfully. In terms of *permanent* weight loss, however, these programs have not always been successful. The question is: Why? What is missing? And what can be done about it?

In *Thin Tastes Better*, Dr. Stephen Gullo answers these questions. For the past twenty years, he has been training obese people to lose weight and keep it off by enabling them to recognize and define their unique "Eating Print." Dr. Gullo uses proven techniques of imaging, repetition of mantras, reinforcement tapes, and scripts. Thus the clients are never alone, so to speak, since they can use their tapes to listen to scripts that reinforce the concepts discussed during their sessions with Dr. Gullo and help them to stay in control.

Dr. Gullo's experience, knowledge, and success are now available in *Thin Tastes Better*. He tells you how to chart the specifics of your Eating Print. Once you do, you will see that you are not out of control with food in general, but only with a few selected foods in very specific situations. "You, and you alone, decide what foods you can and cannot control. You choose the foods that you will abstain from, or limit, or continue to eat without limitations—based on the lessons of your Eating Print, not the arbitrary word of some diet expert."

Uncovering your unique Eating Print is the most liberating and reassuring part of Food Control Training. Dr. Gullo explains how to be in control and how to watch out for your own individual responses. There is no such thing as one diet that works for all people, since the "trigger foods" that lead to relapses and spin you out of control are specific to your Eating Print. The diet plan is a diet plan for life because, as he says, although "you have lost the weight, you have not lost the problem." You must learn from your past history.

The Food Control Eating Plan recommended by Dr. Gullo based on fish, poultry, and a variety of fruits and vegetables is very similar to the diet on which humans evolved. Eating a variety of foods is much healthier than eating a limited number of foods, as most Americans do.

On a temple at Delphi, Socrates' teaching, "Know thyself," was inscribed 2,400 years ago. This philosophy has served humanity well in the past, and now Dr. Gullo has extended this concept to "Know your Eating Print." In helping people understand their uniqueness and the need to be in control of food, Dr. Gullo has adapted the principles of advertising psychology to weight control. This has never been done before, but then again, for many people, attaining a lasting "thin" has never been done before either. It will be interesting to see if the success obtained by Dr. Gullo in helping his clients stay thin can also be accomplished by his book; I think it will.

AN INTRODUCTION TO
FOOD CONTROL TRAINING

If you're holding this book, you probably want to lose weight. More than likely, you've already tried. Perhaps you're one of the millions of Americans who have lost weight on a diet plan, only to gain the pounds back, with interest. Or maybe you've noticed that tightening around the waist when you put on your clothes in the morning and want to stop the expansion before it gets out of hand.

Whatever your situation, you undoubtedly know that the most difficult part of managing your weight isn't *losing* your excess pounds, it's *keeping* them off. Millions of Americans manage to diet away tens of millions of pounds every year—and 95 percent of them gain that weight back.

What has always intrigued me is that elusive 5 percent, the winners of weight control. What do they do? How do they think and feel about food? What do they say to themselves enabling them to overcome the odds that have defeated so many? Those issues have not been effectively scrutinized. By focusing on the majority who "fail," we have missed the opportunity to learn from the minority who succeed—until now.

I have spent years studying the techniques of the winners, and I can say, with absolute assurance, that despite all the depressing statistics, *you can lose weight and keep it off!*

If you've tried to lose weight but found it impossible to stick with a diet plan . . .

If you've lost weight but seen the pounds creep back . . .

Even if you've been heavy for so long that you thought it could never change . . .

You can be thin! Not for weeks, not for months—but for the rest of your life!

I can say this with confidence because my program, Food Control Training, has helped thousands of people achieve and maintain their weight goals. My clients from many countries and many walks of life have conquered their weight problems by learning one simple lesson: *The secret to losing weight is gaining control.*

You too can learn control of the foods, eating patterns, and beliefs about food that prompt you to lose command of what, where, and how much you eat. With Food Control Training, you will learn not only what to eat, but how to manage the food in your life. Not through a fad diet or a quick-fix gimmick, but through a process of self-discovery and self-mastery that identifies the *triggers* that kept you from losing weight in the past and ensures that they will never trip you up again. Food Control Training is your ticket out of the revolving door of weight loss/weight gain.

If you've ever lost weight, somewhere along the way you did something right. If you gained the weight back, somewhere else along the way you did something wrong. Most likely that something was going back to the foods and eating patterns that have been your problem all along. You regained the weight because you lost control of the same foods and the same behaviors—in the very same situations, places, and times of day—that caused you to gain weight in the first place!

We've all heard again and again that diets don't work, but that's not entirely accurate. Diets *alone* don't work. When people follow a diet—by definition, "to eat sparingly according to prescribed rules"—they are putting limits on eating that is out of control. They continue to live within these limits until they reach their desired weight, and then they go off the diet. The control stops when the diet does— and that's the problem.

No one in his right mind purposely loses control and gains back the pounds he worked so hard to lose. No one plans on chronically overeating. If you're like most people, you had every intention of making your weight loss permanent. But somewhere, somehow, something went wrong. Maybe it was at a party, when you spotted a plate of miniature cream puffs. You could almost taste the rich sweetness on your tongue. And so you told yourself the Great Lie of Weight Control: "I'll just have one."

Maybe you did stop at one—that time. But the next day, you remembered your willpower (and the taste) from the night before and thought, "It's okay to have a little once in a while." So you bought yourself a chocolate chip cookie as "a treat." Soon the treats became more frequent, and once you started making exceptions, it became easier and easier to do. Almost before you knew it, you were back to all your old eating patterns—and your old weight.

Sound familiar? It should. I've heard this same story from thousands of clients. For some, the process began with taking a piece of chocolate or a slice of pizza. For others it was bringing home snack foods like pretzels (even "low-fat" ones). For others it was eating when they felt depressed or lonely. Whatever the cause, the end result was the same. One and all, these people were out of control, not because they were weak, ignorant, or self-indulgent, but because they had believed the Great Lie of Weight Control and had fallen victim to the twin threats of *deprivation* and *craving*.

When I meet a new client, I ask if he or she has ever been on a diet before. More than 90 percent say "yes." When I ask what prompted them to slip off their diet, I get all sorts of answers:

"I missed dessert."

"I was tired of feeling punished."

"I missed having my old favorite meals."

"I got tired of the measly portions."

"I couldn't live without ice cream anymore."

"The bread basket was too tempting to pass up."

In different ways, at different times, they all were saying that their diets had collapsed under the weight of deprivation ("I was tired of feeling punished") and/or craving ("It was too tempting to pass up"). Like Scylla and Charybdis, the monsters that crushed passing ships in the Straits of Messina, deprivation and craving have been the undoing of many dieters. Together they tell us that food is the most important thing in the universe and that we should never have to say "no" to any food—no matter how fattening or unhealthy it may be.

It may seem absurd that we can feel deprived in an era when practically every food is just a phone call, walk, or short drive away. Although poverty still exists in our land of plenty, most of us are anything but underfed.

Yet we still feel deprived if we can't have an M&M!

Why? Why is it that when anyone—a doctor, a friend, a loved one—even *hints* that we should limit our food choices, we instantly feel deprived?

The answer can be found in the past—when food *couldn't* be taken for granted. This history of deprivation has been responsible for the "foodification" of modern society. Our culture has become food-centered, food-oriented, and food-glorifying. And because of this most of us have become foodies. It's really no wonder that you've had problems staying on a diet. Diets go against everything you have been programmed to believe about food. *You've been enslaved by food because society is enslaved by food!*

That means everybody, even the "thinnists" of this world—the anorexics, bulimics, waif models, fitness addicts, and so on. They may seem to be the polar opposite of the foodies in outer appearance yet they maintain the very same value system. Both place food before their health and happiness. Whether they crave, overeat, gorge, purge, or spurn that food, it is still food that looms high and mighty in their life, a single abiding obsession.

Deprivation, craving, and our entire foodie culture are like inherited cultural defects. You don't need them. You certainly don't want them. But you've got to deal with them every day.

Dieting alone can't guarantee weight loss. Neither can changing your eating behaviors. No matter what the diet program, no matter how many pounds you lose, the strategies that enabled you to succeed on a diet are not the ones that will work for keeping the weight off. That's why so many people who are adept at losing weight are often inept at keeping it off. You need new strategies for maintaining your healthy weight—strategies that will enable you to stay in control of your eating because the only way to guarantee permanent weight loss is to make permanent changes in your fundamental beliefs about weight and food.

That means developing a whole new model for living with food, a model that frees you from the belief that following a healthy way of eating means deprivation and missing out, one that releases you from the feeling that once you've lost weight you are doomed to an endless struggle to keep it off, one that leaves you feeling liberated, not deprived. It means reaching into your psyche and replacing that ancient internal tape and its messages of deprivation with a new tape filled with positive messages of food control. And it means finding a diet that fits the original Greek meaning of the word, literally, "a manner of living," not a short-term period of eating sparingly, but a long-term plan for eating well and living thin.

The Food Control Training system is the new model you've been looking for. Based on years of listening to what makes people feel deprived on a diet, it deals with the most fundamental feelings experienced by every dieter and enables you to change not only your weight but your head—by rerecording your internal tape and achieving a new, healthy mind-set about food and eating.

Over the years, I have worked with thousands of men and women to successfully change these internal tapes. Their experiences form the backbone of the Food Control Training program. With their help, I have been able to identify the six key steps that will help you make the switch from being *controlled by* food to being *in control of* food.

With these strategies, you will learn that weight control is not a matter of willpower, but *control power*. Control, like a muscle, can be developed and strengthened—not with machines in a gym, but through the winning strategies of Food Control Training.

In this book, I will take you through these strategies step-by-step, guiding you along the path that has brought so many people to their personal, permanent thin. Along the way you will make decisions about what is truly important to you and how much you are willing to do to achieve the goals you set for yourself.

Finally, I will reveal the specifics of the Food Control Eating Plan, a comprehensive approach to living with—and enjoying—food that recognizes the full mosaic of factors that influence eating. This plan has been designed to meet the most fundamental needs of those with weight problems, namely:

- The *psychological and emotional need* for generous servings
- The *tactile need* for foods that are crunchy and creamy
- The *nutritional need* for foods that are high in nutrients while low in fat and calories
- The *practical need* for foods that are convenient, accessible, and easy to prepare

This eating plan is a diet that can guide your food choices to your goal weight and beyond. And it will do it without leaving you feeling deprived or diminished.

Whatever your weight goal, I can guarantee that with Food Control Training you will free yourself from the tyranny of food and the worries of weight. You will know the pleasure of walking up the stairs without running out of breath. You will know the freedom of going out to dinner and not obsessing about the dessert cart. You will know the satisfaction of going to a store and buying the clothes you always wanted and could never wear.

I know this because I have seen it work for so many of the winners at weight loss, winners like Cindy—a woman who had battled obesity for most of her adult life. When she began the Food Control Training program nearly ten years ago, she was nearly 70 pounds overweight. Today she remains within a few pounds of her goal weight of 145 pounds, stopping by my office only once or twice a year for maintenance visits.

On one such visit a few months ago, Cindy came in carrying a dress bag from one of New York's landmark department stores. Gesturing to the bag, she laughed and said, "Do you remember when I could only *dream* of shopping there? The dress in that bag is five sizes smaller than the one I wore the day I first met you! I really can't tell you how grateful I am. If there is ever anything I can ever do for you, I hope you will ask me."

I was touched by Cindy's gratitude, but I pointed out that she, not I, had done all the work and that her success was thanks enough. But as I watched her prepare to leave I had a flash about this book.

"Cindy," I said, "there *is* something you can do for me, if you will. I am writing a book about my weight-control techniques and the people like you who taught them to me. Is there any advice that you would like to give the readers of my book? Specifically, what is it that you say to yourself that enables you to pass up the foods that you once called your goodies, and that tempted you so much?"

Cindy paused a moment and glanced down at the bag at her feet. Then she smiled. "That's easy," she said. "Thin tastes better!"

PART ONE

WHY WE EAT
THE WAY WE DO

OUR CULTURE OF FOOD

*There is small danger of being starved in
our land of plenty; but the danger of being
stuffed is imminent.*
SARAH JOSEPHA HALE

*If an event is meant to matter emotionally,
symbolically, or mystically, food will be
close at hand to sanctify and bind it.*
DIANE ACKERMAN

Over the years, I have learned that it is best not to let people know what I do for a living. No matter what the social occasion, no matter what the original topic of conversation, whenever people learn that I am a "diet doctor" all talk turns to weight and how to lose it. When the nature of my work became known in the community where I have a summer house, I couldn't go to the general store or a restaurant without encountering questions about what foods people should and should not eat. It seems that *everyone* wants to lose weight and no one knows how.

My personal experience is supported by hard economic facts. Every year Americans spend $33 billion on diet programs and products. A few years ago, a major women's magazine polled thirty-three thousand women and discovered the majority would choose losing 10 to 15 pounds as their most desired goal over success in work or love. But despite this national obsession with weight loss, fully one-third of all United States adults over the age of twenty are overweight.

Most discussions of overweight in America focus on *what* Americans are eating—too much fat, too much sugar, too many snacks, etc. But the problem of obesity is far more complex than that.

The epidemic of overweight in America is the product of a complex mosaic of cultural, psychological, and biological factors. Each and every one of these factors exerts a powerful influence on what, why, and how you eat. If you have a weight problem, it may be as much a result of your culture and psychology as it is of your diet and biology.

It is true that for some people the role of biology may be greater than it is for others. But the impact of our cultural psychology is universal. You cannot escape it. When researchers imply that the cure for weight problems will be found in a lab through some magic biological bullet, they are underestimating society's impact. We live in a culture of excess and this excess cannot be cured by any "fat-burning" pills. Even when the precipitating cause for obesity *is* biological, the solution may not be. Because, ultimately, *all* of us must learn to respect the inherent biological limitations of the human body and structure our diets accordingly.

The simple fact is, very few people overeat because of excessive appetite or hunger. Most people overeat (or eat poorly) because easily abused foods are so readily available. We are surrounded by pleasing and tempting foods that can be grabbed in an instant whenever we are bored or upset or the whim strikes us. And we also are surrounded by messages that say "Go ahead, eat it!" regardless of the food's long-term effects. We are victims of cultural psychology and food technology, not biology! Some things won't be cured with a "fat-burning" pill—and cultural programming is one of them. So, if you are serious about permanently changing your weight, it's time to understand—and adjust—your cultural programming.

Food Is Sacred

Food is a link to the past. Every time you sit down to a meal, you are joined by the ghosts of generations of humans for whom every meal was a small victory in an ongoing war against starvation. Getting food was fraught with risk and the possibility of failure. If they wanted a rib roast they had to catch and kill it. They took whatever fruits and vegetables they could find. Sweets (and salt) were rare treats. For our ancestors, food was far more than a taste treat. It was survival. It was prosperity. It was sacred.

Given the hardships associated with getting food, it is small wonder food has always been an integral part of society's festivities. Sometimes there is music, sometimes dancing, at times special prayers or activities, but it is food that raises a gathering from the level of a mere assemblage of people to that of a celebration. The presence of food in abundance means not only survival, but security, status, and the enjoyment of life itself.

For most of history, such abundance was limited to a privileged few. Traditionally, food—and weight—have always meant wealth. When the Earl of Leicester held a banquet in honor of Queen Elizabeth I back in 1575, he served delicacies imported from all over Europe and the "dinner" lasted an incredible seventeen days. Eating in those days was a serious affair. Food was nothing less than a treasure.

But it was a limited treasure. When a medieval serf looked in the larder and said, "There's nothing in the house to eat," he *meant* it. With the dawn of agriculture, food was harvested and stored, but even farming couldn't guarantee a constant food supply. A flood or drought could easily bring want to the most fertile lands—like the devastating potato famine that hit Ireland in 1847. Such famines were responsible for much of the immigration that built this country. And along with their wooden trunks, their customs, and their tales from the Old World, these immigrants brought with them hard-learned lessons of desperation and deprivation, lessons that were reinforced by later periods of want—from the breadlines of the Great Depression to the ration books of World War II. History has taught the people of America to treasure food and do everything in their power to ensure its abundance. And we have learned the lesson well.

Today, although poverty still exists, most Americans live with a prosperity unheard of in human history. We have taken the most exotic dreams and made them as common and attainable as reaching for a pint of Ben & Jerry's Rain Forest Crunch Ice Cream. Everything—and every food—is within our reach.

And, good children of starving immigrants that we are, we are reaching all the time. The idea of avoiding a food— particularly a pleasurable one—is antagonistic to everything we believe in. We worked for it, we deserve it, and so we are going to eat it. The threat that in doing so we may destroy our health as well as our appearance isn't strong enough to offset the immediate gratification of satisfying whatever dietary whim comes along. We have become a "foodie" society—food-centered and food-glorifying.

You only need look around the landscape (or the television dial) to see how we worship food. Our "temples" are twenty-four-hour, wide-aisled, freeway-style supermarkets and "family-style" restaurants where tables groan under the weight of piles of food. From sea to shining sea, we live according to the bylaws of foodie-ism:

Food is success!
Food is reward!
Food is joy!
Food is relief from boredom!
Food is consolation!
Food is celebration!

Above all, food is sacred. Too sacred to be limited now that it is finally available in such abundance.

Happiness (or so we're led to believe) is never having to say "no" to the foods that symbolize survival, satisfaction, and success. The perfect diet is one that will allow us to be thin while never refusing any food. We keep our cupboards stocked with far more food than we could eat in a month, never mind a week. Food is important, we tell ourselves, and we deserve to have it in abundance. Because food not only feeds the body, it feeds the soul.

Food Is Comfort

For many nationalities and ethnic groups, food means more than survival and wealth; it also means comfort. From the stereotypical Jewish or Italian grandmother to the most lavish southern hostess, the implicit message behind all meals is: "Eat, you'll feel better!"

You can probably remember times when your mother or grandmother said much the same thing to you as she proffered a plate of cookies or a bowl of hot soup. The amazing thing was you probably *did* feel better after those cookies or that bowl of soup. It was during childhood, when things *could* be made right with a cookie, that many of us learned to appreciate, desire, *need* the specific foods we turn to as adults. From cookies to buttered popcorn to homemade biscuits hot from the oven, these "comfort foods" resonate on both physical and emotional levels.

Comfort foods vary according to our family history, ethnic background, and cultural traditions, which is why your cultural background is as important as your individual history in understanding your control problems with food. Is it surprising that a girl from Louisiana, brought up in her grandmother's kitchen on the banks of the Mississippi, fueled by fried crawfish and cream of artichoke and shrimp soup, rich gumbo ya ya and sticky sweet pralines, would have a strong desire for foods with that fatty appeal? Yet that now grown-up woman in New Orleans ignores the obvious environmental pressures and blames herself when she is not at her desired weight.

The same goes for the Texan, with his chicken-fried steak, his pan-handle-sized biscuits, and every meal swimming in brown gravy. The food preferences and comfort foods of people are conditioned by the cultures that produce them. And whatever your background, you have received some sort of conditioning as well, conditioning that leads you to prefer the special foods that were given to you as rewards for grand accomplishments or as consolation when you were feeling blue.

Consider Andrew, a Wall Street banker who was hooked on Twizzlers for years before he thought back to where his love of licorice began. He recalled the spelling bees held every Friday in his grammar school. Every time he won, his father would take him down to the candy store and award him a prize of licorice.

Or Marjorie, who developed her passion for ice cream

back when she was on the varsity tennis team. Her mother would pick up Marjorie and her girlfriends after every match and, to rouse their spirits, treat them all to ice cream cones on the days when they lost—which were many. Win or lose, food made the event.

Who does not have memories of this kind? After all, the first expressions of love and affection that we receive are given when we are fed. Mother's milk, rich in nutrients and antibodies, serves both as food and a sort of epidemiologic memory. We are nourished not only by the food but by the warmth, the stroking, the sense of security we receive.

PEOPLE ARE TALKING ABOUT . . .

Even our language is teeming with proof of our obsession with food. Look up *taste* in the dictionary and you'll find it linked to critical judgment, discernment, and a fine appreciation of life, whereas something tasteless is dull and uninteresting and in bad taste refers to something vulgar. To *lick* is to overcome, beat, or conquer—and getting in one's licks is to grab an opportunity. A hard worker earns his "daily *bread,*" or is shown to be "worth his *salt,*" which is, interestingly enough, where the word *salary* comes from. Even the word *companion* originally referred to someone with whom one shared bread.

What are our terms of endearment? "Honey," "cookie," "sweetie." How do we describe a particularly gorgeous woman? "Luscious," "delicious," "a real dish." Shapely females pose for "cheesecake" photos, male models for "beefcake" shots.

In Paris, a woman may call her lover *mon petit chou* ("my little cabbage"). In Britain, a sweetheart is a "crumpet." And if she's caught playing around, the *sweet*heart sours into a "tart." Even in Ghana, the verb "to eat" is used by certain tribes when referring to sex, the expressions of food and love blending until they are indistinguishable.

WHITE AND GREEN ✦ WHITE IS LIGHT, GREEN IS LEAN ✦ IF YOU ARRIVE

Flash forward to years later. You're up late, channel surfing with the TV remote, and through the din of infomercials, Nick at Night reruns, and music videos comes a familiar voice: "Frosted Flakes . . . they're grrrrreat!" Tony the Tiger? At this hour? You may have wondered why "kids' stuff" like this is on when the kids are asleep. But advertisers know, even if adults do not, the valuable memories these foods hold.

Sure, food tastes good, and that's certainly part of the reason why we eat too much. But it's also history, our personal history, our innermost traditions. When you bite into a muffin or a cookie or even a peanut butter and jelly sandwich, you are engaging in "retro eating." Your brain reacts to tastes and smells so quickly, helping you recall the past like nothing else can.

Women and the Specter of Weight

Open up any women's magazine and you won't have to turn many pages before you hit an article on anorexia or bulimia. Millions of women suffer—and some die—from eating disorders. Here is prime evidence that weight consciousness in our time is wreaking havoc on a significant portion of society. The twentieth century marked the dawn of a new era—suddenly, thin was in, and like never before. Headlines, billboard images, and articles in women's magazines proclaimed it. But it wasn't always like this.

Prior to World War I, women's bodies struck much fuller silhouettes. The ideal woman was buxom, round, fleshy. Myths passed down for thousands of years extolled the virtues of such ample women, women like Gaia, who created the galaxies by pouring milk from her breasts. The full-figured feminine image was honored in countless paintings by artists like Rubens and Botticelli. Statues of

Venus, still standing today, reflect the beauty norms of the past: sloping bellies, hillocks of thighs, layers of maternal comfort, and womanhood.

But after the Great War, doughboys returned home from the front to find that the female silhouette had changed. Gone were the curves formed by bosom and corset and petticoat. Thin was "in" primarily due to shortages of flour, sugar, and other food staples used in the war. Fashion styles changed, too, when the modern-day girdle arrived on the scene (replacing the cumbersome corset) and streamlined and casual looks like dropped waists and flapper dresses became the rage. Women not only danced the Charleston till dawn but took up fitness activities in greater numbers than ever before. Though a slightly more voluptuous look would regain popularity in the 1930s, 1940s, and 1950s (remember Lana Turner, Jane Russell, Marilyn Monroe), the food limitations for women eventually resumed—this time, however, not induced by war rations or shortages.

Instead the modern frenzy for thin was and continues to be driven by the fashion industry (which creates clothing that looks best on the rail thin). It is prodded by the models and celebrities seen in the media. And, worst of all, it is encouraged—or at least tolerated—by ourselves.

Reality Check

Women today are faced with a struggle. Contradictory messages concerning food and weight have been around for at least two thousand years, probably longer. In previous centuries, Japanese women were expected to eat out of smaller rice bowls and use shorter, slimmer chopsticks. In China, though the women of the imperial court were allowed to host banquets, they were segregated from the men and were offered fewer courses and less wine than their male counterparts.

At many feasts during the Middle Ages, European noblemen were invited to dine; noblewomen, on the other hand, were expected to sit in a reserved balcony and observe. And in this century, when it was common throughout Europe to find several families living in one dwelling, the dinner ritual would be that the men ate first, the women served. You name it—any century, any culture—women have been expected, in general, to be surrounded by food and at the same time cordon themselves off from it. This history, combined with wildly diverging definitions of the ideal body type, is enough to confuse anyone.

The contradictions of yesterday are so inbred that a modern woman of the '90s still can't evaluate her own body accurately. Current research proves that women are more likely than men to perceive themselves as overweight regardless of their actual weight. One study projected that the total number of women in this country who are overweight comes to 46 percent—but 75 percent of women who look at themselves in the mirror *think* they are! Other studies show that women suffer from eating disorders significantly more than men and have lower levels of body satisfaction and self-esteem.

Since the 1960s, *Playboy* centerfolds have become increasingly slender, as have beauty pageant contestants. Over this time period, the weight of the average woman has risen, but the weight she desires for herself has diminished. In fact, studies show that a majority of women maintain images of their ideal body that are significantly skinnier than the image most men, and even most women, find attractive in others.

The cruelest twist of all is that the role models themselves, the fashion models who parade their wraithlike bodies on the covers of national magazines, are not even as skinny as they appear. Look at any cover model and you'll see not God's handiwork but the Scitex touch. The Scitex, that modern miracle of publishing, is a machine that airbrushes and alters photos so an editor can create virtually any look she wants for a model. For every cover, hips are trimmed, busts enlarged, stomachs flattened. The wrinkles vanish, lips become pinker, fuller, eyes bluer, hair blonder. "We correct the little imperfections," an editor might say. And what does the woman at the checkout stand think as she looks at an array of these fictional images? "Why can't I look like *them?*"

And women aren't the only ones making this plea. Men also are being objectified and sexualized in movies, ads, and art. Madison Avenue, Hollywood, and television present male images of engorged limbs, honed to perfection by hours of work with personal trainers and makeup artists. And men seeing these images say, "I don't *look* like that."

Women have been saying that to themselves for ages and they have the eating disorders to prove it. But up to 5 percent of those with food disorders are men. And their numbers are likely to increase as the images and physical expectations of men change and become more unattainable.

The Bottom Line

The past forty years have seen a drastic shift in the way we eat. From "plate eaters," who consumed meat-and-potatoes meals while sitting at the family table, we have become "snack eaters," consuming food on the run, relying on high-starch, high-fat snack foods that provide neither the social nor nutritional satisfaction that human well-being demands. These foods are available at all times in unlimited amounts and appeal to the most basic of our cultural food instincts—make it quick and easy, and never say no.

At the same time, the old societal ideal of "weight means wealth" has been replaced by the new ideal of "thin is in." It's a formula for disaster, and the disaster is becoming more and more clear. We are suffering from a cultural neurosis—torn between conflicting belief systems and values, and growing fatter and more distressed by the day.

If you're worried or think all is lost, remember one simple truth: *Mind-sets are changeable.* It's like a tape recorder inside your head. It doesn't matter if the tape is two thousand years old *(Food is sacred!)* or only eighty *(Thin is in!)*.

With the skills of Food Control Training, you can change that tape.

Why am I so sure? Food Control Training is the only weight-control program in the world that points out the societal programming in your life, that respects its power, and that teaches you techniques to overcome it.

I'm not saying it's easy. It takes work. But it can be done.

So if you're really interested in controlling your weight, if you really want to master the foods that trip you up time and again, if you really want to lose pounds, first drop two thousand. No, not pounds. Years. You'll be amazed at how much less needy you'll feel and how much thinner you'll be.

WHY YOU LOVE
THE FOODS YOU DO

*Since shortages from mild to severe were
absolutely ubiquitous for humans, natural
selection obviously favors individuals who
can store calories in times of surplus. We
are stocking up for a famine that never
comes.*
MELVIN KONNER

*Three million years ago, Mother Nature
had no way of knowing that one day
cheesecake would be invented.*
WILLIAM BENNETT, M.D., AND JOEL GURIN

Joanna walked briskly into my office and dropped into the
wing-backed chair facing my desk, a look of frustration and
amusement on her face.

"I'm going to kill my husband!" she announced, leaning
forward. "Or at least I'm going to divorce him. . . . Then
again, maybe I'll just never eat another meal with him again
as long as I live."

"What did he do?" I asked.

"It's not what he *does,*" she replied. "It's what he *doesn't*
do! We were just at lunch, and there was a chocolate

mousse cake on the dessert menu. Now, you know how I am with chocolate . . . so I had some fresh fruit. But Doug ordered the cake and when it came—looking just glorious—he had two, maybe three bites and then he *pushed it away!*" She shook her head in amazement. "Can you believe it? Where does he get so much self-control?"

Joanna had just come face to face with one of life's most central truths: Tastes differ—between men and women, between individuals, even between ethnic groups. Doug doesn't necessarily have more self-control than Joanna, he just doesn't share her sweet tooth. He's a salt fiend—if it's coated in salt, he'll eat it. Doug's physician has been trying to get him to cut back on salt for years, and Doug freely admits that it's a major battle.

Cultural and psychological influences are only part of the story of individual food preferences and cravings, or *differential food preferences.* The external pressures and psychology of deprivation that influence what we put in our mouths are matched by equally powerful *internal* forces. We carry a biology of deprivation that is rooted in our genes, gender, and individual biochemistry.

Why Fat Is Hard to Fight

The most basic goal of every living creature is survival and the most basic requirement for survival is energy—in the form of calories taken in from food.

In order to survive in the harsh conditions that have existed for most of human history, the human body had to find a way to make the most of food when food was abundant, so that it could keep going when food was scarce. It achieved this goal in two ways: *energy storage* and *energy conservation.* When there are a lot of calories in the diet, the body uses what it needs and stores the rest in fat cells.

When calories are cut back, the body conserves energy by slowing down its energy burning processes, or metabolism.

Ideally, your body would draw on the calories stored in your fat cells any time you reduced your caloric intake. But like an investor who doesn't want to withdraw any principal, the body "sees" its fat cells as the last resort in the fight against starvation. It is quick to make deposits into the fat bank but very slow to make withdrawals. And it is this basic biological fact that poses such a problem for modern humans—particularly modern humans who want to lose weight.

Many scientists suggest that whenever you try to lose weight by severely cutting back on calories—particularly if the cutback is drastic—your body sees the caloric reduction as a famine. It responds by going into survival mode. It slows down the basic processes of day-to-day living—the Resting Metabolic Rate (RMR)—and draws on the body's tissues to get some of the additional energy (calories) it believes it needs. Unfortunately, it doesn't turn to the fat cells for that extra energy. Instead, it first breaks down some of your *muscle* tissue—and that's bad.

Muscle cells, unlike fat cells, are active; they actually work. The mitochondria of muscle cells are like little energy plants—they are responsible for burning many of the calories we take in each day. The more muscle tissue you have, the more efficiently you burn calories. Conversely, when you lose muscle tissue, you lose some of your body's ability to burn calories. When the body uses up muscle tissue to compensate for the "starvation" of dieting, it accomplishes two tasks at once. It gets extra energy but it also slows down your metabolism.

The fact is, you can't trick your body into becoming permanently thin by temporarily depriving it of food. It's too smart to fall into that trap. It is the descendant of millions of other bodies that survived true starvation—famines far worse than anything you could impose while on a diet. As far as your body is concerned, it has one job: to keep alive and to keep those fat cells filled up and ready for the next time the food supply runs out. And there is some evidence that the more you diet, the better your body gets at its job.

Research suggests that when a diet is stopped, the body—believing it has just endured a minifamine—gets to work restoring the status quo, plus interest. When a dieter goes back to "normal" eating, the body starts packing the calories away into the fat cells once again, often with a little extra, just in case. Dieting tells the body that the world is a dangerous place where food can become scarce at any time, so it had better hoard those calories and conserve as much energy as possible. What this lesson means in the long run is still a subject of some debate. Some scientists believe that the metabolic downshift is permanent, but a recent analysis of the scientific research indicates that this may not be the case. Although the jury is still out, one thing is clear—drastic dieting doesn't work. If you want to reach a healthy weight and *stay* there, you need to do it at a reasonable pace, and work within the limitations and needs of your biology.

Maybe someday the human race will evolve beyond the biology of deprivation and the human body will stop stocking up for a famine that never comes. In previous centuries, people died from too little food. Today, in our culture of excess and foodie-ism, we are dying from too much food. In the long run, therefore, obesity actually works against the basic survival instinct of the human body. But evolution is slow. If you want to lose weight today, in this human body, you have to accept and respect the lessons of evolution. This means *not* falling for get-thin-quick schemes that reduce your calorie intake to next to nothing. It also means developing an understanding of how—and why—your body responds to certain foods.

Making Food Work for You: The Thermogenic Effect

In nature, most foods come in complicated "packages" that the body must undo before it can get to the calories and nutrients inside. Simply taking a food into your mouth doesn't always mean that you are getting nourishment into your cells. In order for that to happen, your body has to break the food down into its component parts through digestion and then absorb and process those parts for distribution and use by the body's cells.

This process takes energy, and the amount of energy required for the breakdown of any given food is called its *thermogenic effect.* The thermogenic effect is an indicator of how many calories the body must use to process and store the food we eat. The remaining calories are either used to fuel the body's life processes (including the RMR) or stored as fat. The greater a food's thermogenic effect, the less likely it is that there will be calories left over for storage.

Of the three primary food types—protein, fat, and carbohydrates—both protein and carbohydrates are thermogenic. Each contains about 4 calories per gram and the body must literally rev itself up to break down these foods and put their nutrients and calories to use. Researchers at the University of Lausanne in Switzerland have estimated that for every 100 calories of protein we consume, the body uses 25 to 40 calories during thermogenesis. Similarly, for every

100 calories of carbohydrate—specifically glucose—the body uses 6 to 8 calories.

Fat—which at 9 calories per gram is far more calorically dense than protein and carbohydrate—has almost no thermogenic effect. In fact, for every 100 calories of fat you consume, the body uses only 3 calories in thermogenesis! And unlike protein and carbohydrates, the body has no mechanism for revving itself up when fat intake goes up. Instead of working harder, the body shunts extra dietary fat straight into storage. So if you've ever said that ice cream "goes straight to my hips," you weren't too far off the mark.

Although protein is the most thermogenic food element, many of the better protein sources are also high in fat, which is why so many physicians and nutritionists advise their clients to steer clear of beef, pork, and other protein foods. To take full advantage of the thermogenic effect of protein, it is important to choose low-fat protein sources such as fish, legumes, and poultry. This is why I call seafood and fish—not carbohydrates—the Concorde to thin.

Just as not all protein sources are created equal, not all carbohydrates are created equal. And although carbohydrates do indeed make up the bulk of the human diet, choosing the right carbohydrates is a very important part of weight loss and maintenance.

Understanding Carbohydrates

The term *carbohydrates* covers a lot of territory. Lettuce is a carbohydrate. So is broccoli. But so is a loaf of white bread, or a teaspoon of sugar, or a dry martini on the rocks. A carbohydrate is anything that can be broken down into the simple sugar that our cells use. What distinguishes one group of carbs from another is their level of complexity—

how easily they are broken down by the body and reduced to blood glucose.

When it comes to converting food into blood sugar, however, faster and easier isn't necessarily better. Your cells need to have a steady, reliable fuel supply, and the body's been equipped with a marvelous system of checks and balances that keeps blood sugar levels as constant as possible. People used to eat lots of raw (or at least fresh) vegetables and fruits, an occasional bit of meat, and—on very rare occasions—some type of concentrated sweet, like honey. When humans began farming, the amount of meat and milk products increased and, not surprisingly, so did the percentage of fat in the diet; but the basic staples of fruits, vegetables, and relatively whole grains (like wheat) stayed pretty much the same. The body knew how to handle these foods; it had been doing it for quite a while.

Then humans discovered how to make two substances that would change the food supply forever. During the eighteenth century we learned how to strip wheat and other grains of their hard outer shells and nutritious inner "germ" and refine them down into exceptionally fine flours. At around the same time, sugar became a major part of the human diet (and economy). It was not long before white flour and sugar became dietary staples for anyone who could afford them. Today sugar (in its various forms) has become so ubiquitous that the average American eats more than 125 pounds a year!

Insulin—The Hunger Hormone

The most important of the body's mechanisms for controlling glucose is a hormone called insulin. Produced by specialized cells in the pancreas, insulin is released into the bloodstream whenever blood sugar levels rise. Its job is to get sugar out of the bloodstream and pack it into the cells. When blood glucose levels rise—such as when you're at a buffet enjoying the *baba au rhum*—the pancreas responds by pouring insulin into the bloodstream. The insulin rushes through the body, pushing sugar into the cells. But your cells can hold only so much, and when they can't accept any more, insulin helps the body convert the excess sugar into fat—and not just any fat but the very forms that are most associated with arterial disease and heart attacks, including cholesterol.

Once the levels of blood sugar have been reduced—either through delivery to the cells or conversion to fat—the body is left with something of a dilemma. There is still insulin circulating in the bloodstream, looking for work. But now the blood sugar level has dropped. So the body sends out another message: "Get me some more sugar!" You experience that message as an increase in appetite. If you respond to the message with another piece of cake, the cycle will start all over again.

You've probably already gone through this cycle—when you've had sweet-and-sour chicken with white rice for dinner and felt hungry an hour later, or when you've had a candy bar to "take the edge off" your midafternoon hunger and realized you were ravenous again within twenty minutes. Insulin is truly the hunger hormone, and when you persistently eat foods that prompt your body to oversecrete insulin—that is, when you eat foods that are high in sugar or refined carbohydrates like white flour—*you are programming your body to be more hungry more of the time!*

Don't blame your body for this state of affairs. It doesn't know that there is an all-night supermarket right down the block. It thinks you are always in imminent danger of starvation. Your body wants only what is best for your survival.

CAN "GOOD FOODS" MAKE YOU HUNGRY?

For years I have observed that many of my clients seem most likely to lose control of their eating when relying on starchy carbohydrate foods—even supposedly "good" foods like bagels or pastas. From a food control perspective, the answer to the problem is fairly simple: Limit those foods. But it presents a much more interesting clinical dilemma. What is it about these clients' physiology that makes them so susceptible to some carbohydrates?

The answer came only recently, in the form of research conducted by Drs. Richard and Rachael Heller of the Mount Sinai School of Medicine in New York City. The Hellers evaluated the insulin response of normal and overweight adults and discovered something truly remarkable. When given identical doses of glucose during a glucose tolerance test, overweight and normal weight subjects showed dramatically different patterns of insulin release. In the overweight subjects, insulin levels rose dramatically, causing glucose to be removed from the bloodstream at an accelerated rate. Within an hour or two of the test, the overweight subjects had very low blood sugar levels and very high circulating insulin levels. The result? They felt hungry!

This phenomenon has a lot to do with why saying "I'll just have a little" or "just this once" may not work for you. And why the classic weight-control dogma—that once you lose the weight, you will be able to moderate certain foods—may be working against your own biology. It was my own clients who taught me this when, in the maintenance stage of Food Control Training, they told me, "Now that it's out of my life, I don't want to have it back in my life because the cravings and my problems will return. A little only leads to more and more."

To reach a healthy weight and stay there, you have to get beyond the tyranny of your taste buds and use your *mind*, not your appetite, to make food choices. Remember, in our modern world of overabundance, the taste buds don't know what they are talking about. That's why it is particularly dangerous for people to live their lives guided by their taste buds rather than good judgment.

This raises another rather sticky question: When it comes to nutrition, just what is good judgment?

"Nutritionally Correct" Versus "Weight-Control Correct"

Nutrition is a young science, and much of what we know in this field was discovered only in the last half century. But you'd never know that from some of the confident pronouncements and nutritional advice that is regularly doled out to the public. The fact is, the "nutritionally correct" advice that you hear on the radio and television may not be "weight-control correct" or suited to your individual needs.

For several years now, the nutritionally correct guide for making food choices has been the United States Department of Agriculture's (USDA) Food Guide Pyramid. This multitiered guide states that the foundation of every dietary plan should be grain foods such as breads, pastas, and rice. The reason? The high nutrient and fiber content of most whole grains. Unfortunately, this nutritionally correct advice fails on several counts as a guide for those who want to lose weight.

- First and foremost, most nutritional research is based not on overweight subjects, but on normal weight students, patients, and volunteers. The nutritional needs— and biological reactions—of these individuals are markedly different from those of people with weight problems.
- Second, many of the "grain foods" listed at the base of the USDA pyramid are in fact *flour* foods—pastas and breads made from refined flours that have none of the

nutritional benefits of whole grains. What they *do* have plenty of is calories and the refined carbohydrates that can elevate blood sugar and prompt the release of insulin, the hunger hormone.

- Finally, and perhaps most important, there is the problem of the USDA's serving-size fantasy. According to the USDA, you should have six to eleven servings from the bread, cereal, rice, and pasta group every day. What's a serving? A single slice of bread or a mere $\frac{1}{2}$ *cup* of cooked pasta, cereal, rice, or other grain. When was the last time you ate a half cup of cooked pasta? Most restaurants serve four times that amount in a single entrée. For most overweight individuals, a half-cup serving of anything is certain to trigger a (rather understandable!) sense of deprivation—precisely the thing they want to avoid.

From a control perspective, therefore, grains and grain-based foods are the worst possible foundation for a dietary plan. And it is for this reason that my program calls for far less grains, cereals, and flour-based foods. Instead, it looks to research that has been conducted on people with weight problems and to a much older set of dietary guidelines—the eating habits of our hunter-gatherer ancestors.

Learning from Evolution

The human body was designed a long time before supermarkets dotted the landscape or even before grains were cultivated. In fact, the human body was designed at a time when the most abundant foods were plants and an occasional animal carcass. This hunter-gatherer eating pattern persisted for a good portion of human history. It was only in the last century that the Big Three of fat, flour, and sugar

WHATEVER HAPPENED TO THE 200-CALORIE BAGEL?

Have you ever wondered how many calories are in your healthy, low-fat morning bagel? What about that slice of pizza you had for lunch? If you think the U.S. Department of Agriculture is the place to ask, think again. Calorie counts in the real world and calorie counts in the official realm of the USDA have very little to do with each other.

According to the USDA, the average bagel—without butter or cream cheese—contains about 200 calories. But a recent study conducted by the *New York Times* found that the USDA's estimate is off—way off. In fact, when the *Times* had nutritional analyses run on twenty bagels bought at a variety of shops around New York City, they found that the average calorie count was more than *twice* the USDA's estimate! The lowest-calorie bagel had 307 calories and the highest-calorie bagel had a whopping 552 calories.

A few months after its bagel exposé, the *Times* went after another favorite food—pizza. The USDA's pizza profile describes a 2-ounce slice with 140 calories and 3.21 grams (29 calories) of fat. But on the streets of New York (and at a couple of national chains) the average pizza slice was twice that size, with twice as many calories and three times as much fat. In fact, one pizzeria had a "healthy" slice that weighed in at $10^1/2$ ounces, 610 calories, and *17 grams of fat!*

The serving sizes and calorie counts touted by the government were undoubtedly accurate at one time, but in today's world of "more is better" the 140-calorie pizza slice and 200-calorie bagel have gone the way of the dinosaur and dodo bird.

became a staple of the human diet. And with them came a remarkable rise in heart disease, diabetes, cancer, and other diseases that some researchers call "the diseases of civilization."

Today, nutrition researchers from around the world are taking a closer look at older, more traditional diets, and they are discovering an interesting pattern. Societies that consume diets rich in vegetables, low-fat protein sources (such as seafood), and truly *whole* grains have much lower disease rates than those with diets high in fat, flour, and sugar products. Scientists such as Artemis Simopoulos, M.D., president of the Center for Genetics, Nutrition and Health in Washington, D.C., and the elite team at the Harvard School of Public Health and the Oldways Preservation Trust are on the cutting edge of research that could change not only the way we eat, but how long (and how well) we will live. These creative thinkers have gone beyond the confines of the lab to examine the lessons of history and the human experience. And with each new finding, it becomes more and more clear that the most healthful diet is not that of the USDA's Food Guide Pyramid. Even more importantly, from a control perspective, a diet that may be healthful for your neighbor could well spell disaster for you—depending on your individual food preferences.

Understanding Cravings: The Preferential Food Response

Just as there are variations in the basic human body type, so there are variations in our preferences and responses to food. Some of these preferential food responses seem to be genetically influenced—inherited from our parents, grandparents, and so on. Others are learned as we are exposed to various foods. Although most humans will exhibit some preference for the Big Three—sugar, flour, fat—the strength and specificity of those preferences can vary quite a bit from person to person.

For many, two very powerful taste preferences—for sweet and for salt—seem to be present almost from birth.

The natural attraction to salty and sweet foods can be enhanced by increased exposure to them, particularly when that exposure starts young. Babies who are given sugary liquids will consume increasing amounts of liquid when the concentration of sugar is increased. Similar results have been obtained with salty solutions in both human and animal experiments. So the more you were exposed to a particular high-risk taste early in life (and for many of us, it starts in those first few days in the hospital when babies are often nourished with a 5-percent glucose solution), the more you will be attracted to it in your later years. If you have children, think about that the next time you're in the supermarket and they are clamoring for junk food. The lessons of genetics indicate that your children may very well end up with a weight problem just like yours, especially if you start feeding them the very foods that set you on the road to overweight.

The preferential food response often appears to be a classic conditioned response to specific food cues. Like Pavlov's dogs salivating at the sound of a bell they associate with food, the human body learns to set various biochemical events in motion the minute it experiences certain tastes. In some people, for example, the taste of artificial sweeteners may prompt a release of insulin into the bloodstream, even though these sweeteners have none of the biological components of real sugar. As a result, the mere sensation of sweetness, be it real or artificial, triggers an increase in appetite! That means you may find yourself eating more diet candies than you ever intended.

This doesn't mean, however, that artificial sweeteners cannot help you. For many men and women they help to control the desire for high-fat, high-calorie sweets. Once again, the message is clear: Watch out for your own indi-

vidual responses, for there is no such thing as one diet that
works for all people.

This kind of conditioning is not limited to foods that are
sweet or salty. *Any* food that is perceived as especially
palatable and rewarding can trigger a reaction in the same
brain circuits that are activated by stimulant drugs. Foods
with "mouth feel" seem to be particularly potent. For example:

- *Crunchy foods* like potato chips and pretzels seem ex-
  pressly designed to foster uncontrolled eating. My
  clients consistently place crunchy foods (especially
  flour-based products) high on their list of foods that increase their appetites. There is also some research evidence that the sound and muscular action of chewing
  crunchy foods has a stress-relieving effect, making
  them all the more attractive to people who eat when
  they are under stress.
- *Creamy foods,* such as ice cream and mashed potatoes,
  tend to be among the most comforting foods, partly because they are so often high in fat (which tends to have
  a slightly sedating effect) and partly because the texture is so evocative of childhood.

Individual differences in neurochemistry—the chemical
behavior of the brain—have a tremendous effect on the
types of foods we prefer and crave, much to the chagrin of
some scientists. For years, folk remedies relied on food to
relieve everything from the common cold to sleeplessness
to just feeling tense; and for years many scientists said that
food couldn't possibly change your mood—that food's influence on the brain was limited to blood glucose. Then
several groups of researchers showed that other compo-

nents of food, particularly the amino acids tryptophan and tyrosine, could actually cross the blood-brain barrier and change the chemical functioning of the brain.

Tryptophan, an amino acid present in large amounts in dairy foods, turkey, and many starchy carbohydrates like potatoes, is a building block of serotonin—one of the chemicals that brain cells use to communicate and that helps regulate mood. So eating foods high in tryptophan tends to have a calming effect. Think how you feel after eating a hefty meal like Thanksgiving dinner. It's no coincidence that everyone feels a little drowsy and relaxed; that's serotonin at work. In fact, it has been suggested that people who crave carbohydrates are actually craving these calming effects of serotonin. Tyrosine, on the other hand, which is concentrated in many protein foods, tends to have an energizing effect.

These findings are only the beginning. There is much to learn about the neurochemical effects of food and the physiology of food preferences and cravings. Food is much more than an energy source for the body, and individual food preferences are more than just passing whims. That's why mastering the skills of Food Control Training is so important: They enable you to control your food preferences instead of being controlled by them. Food Control Training teaches you to use your body as your textbook—to listen to how it responds to food, not only at the time you eat it, but also hours (or even days) later.

Why Women Gain Weight Faster Than Men

If you are a woman, you're already aware of what one of my clients has called "life's cruelest joke": Women gain weight faster and lose weight more slowly than men. I wish that I could say this was a myth, but I can't. It's true.

The reason is simple. Women get pregnant; men don't. And by that I don't just mean that women gain weight when they have babies. They do, of course, and since fat tends to attract fat, even a relatively small postpregnancy weight gain can have a tremendous additive effect over time. But there's more to it than that.

At any given moment, a woman of childbearing age needs to have enough stored energy reserves to meet not only her basic physiological needs, but those of a growing baby—both in and out of the womb. How did nature provide for this eventuality? It made the female body exceptionally good at turning calories into fat, and even better at holding onto that fat. Just look at the biological statistics:

- Women have more fat cells, bigger fat cells, and more of the enzymes that help store that fat than men.
- Men have more of the enzymes that burn fat.
- Women have estrogen, the primary female hormone, which seems to send this fat particularly to the lower body for storage where it's extra tough to burn off.
- Men have more testosterone, which sends fat to the abdominal region.
- Women have a generally lower metabolism.
- Men have more muscle mass, which actively burns calories.

So a diet that will work for a man could provide far too many calories for a woman, even if they are the same height and have the same overall activity level.

Women, effectively "programmed" to maintain more fat cells, may also be more likely to crave foods that will feed those fat cells, particularly sugar and fat. And the monthly variations in hormone levels, which signal the body to prepare for an impending pregnancy, also affect the nature and strength of food cravings. Most women experience an increase in appetite in the days around their menstrual cycle, and the majority of those are struck by very powerful, specific cravings. While diets (and dieters) that ignore these cyclic changes in cravings do so at their peril, my eating plan specifically adjusts the menu to meet this biological need in women.

Why Men Should Worry

The biological statistics are not entirely stacked in men's favor. Women tend to accumulate fat in their buttocks and thighs, the so-called pear shape. Men usually store fat around the abdomen, the apple shape. Research has shown that people with the apple type of fat distribution are at much higher risk of high blood cholesterol, stroke, heart disease, high blood pressure, and diabetes, perhaps because the fat that accumulates around the abdomen (brown fat) is thought to be more "active" than the white fat that typically builds up in the lower body and may enhance the production of LDL (or "bad") cholesterol. So, male or female, if you are apple shaped, it is particularly important for you to slim down!

Smart Dieters, Foolish Choices

Every day you are surrounded by foods that—thanks to evolution—you have been designed to prefer, to enjoy, to crave. But there is good news: The same biology that got you into this situation can also get you out of it. You've also inherited a large, well-developed brain capable of making intelligent, reasoned decisions based on more than the impulses of your taste buds.

IT'S NOT A MOUNTAIN TO CLIMB, IT'S JUST A FEW PATTERNS TO MASTER

Food preferences *can* be overcome and relearned. In fact, when people avoid high-fat or high-sugar foods, they start to lose their taste for these foods within only a few months. Your mind and body can work together to make it easier for you to eat properly and well, if you learn and practice the necessary skills. And the longer you do it, the easier it gets.

The only problem is, if you go *back* to these foods on a regular basis—even in small amounts—the old preferences tend to resurface. This is why those who say, "Have a little, so you don't feel deprived" are often being naïve. Many of my clients who abstained from certain foods while losing weight discovered that whenever they went back to the occasional sweet, or bread, or other flour product that caused trouble in the past, they weren't satisfied but constantly hungry . . . and craving these foods.

Biology is not destiny. If you keep your body well-nourished with the *right* foods, you won't feel such intense cravings for the wrong ones.

More than forty years ago, researchers at the University of Texas at Austin showed how animals lacking proper nourishment tend to make inept food choices. The researchers observed a group of malnourished and stressed lab animals. When the animals were given a choice among food, water, or an alcohol/water solution, they showed a marked preference for the alcohol mixture. (Alcohol may be the ultimate refined carbohydrate, since it contains nothing but calories.) The more malnourished these animals were, the more they seemed to seek out simple calories, even when given access to healthy food. In the words of one of the researchers, the animals seemed to lose their inherent "wisdom of the body." Weakened and stressed, they could only seek out the quickest fix available. When the animals were no longer stressed, their preference changed once again. Instead of going for the alcohol solution, the animals went for food and plain water. Their "wisdom of the body" was restored.

What does this have to do with humans? Although it is true that many (if not most) Americans are overweight, it is also true that a good number of them are malnourished. Most Americans take in plenty of calories (usually in the form of snack and fast foods), but not nearly enough vitamins, minerals, and other nutrients. Too many of us have lost our "wisdom of the body" and seek out the wrong foods.

No authority or textbook can replace the information you get from your own body. The nutritional truths of today are often the myths of tomorrow. Only a few decades ago all calories were considered equal. Today we are just beginning to unravel the complexities of thermogenesis and metabolism. In the 1970s and '80s starch was considered the root of all weight problems. In the 1990s fat has become the culprit. These are just a few examples of nutritional ideas that were proven facts in one decade and proven folly in the next.

When it comes to weight loss and food control, let your body—and your history—be your guide. If a textbook or doctor says you can eat something and you find yourself gaining weight or losing control, that food's not for you, no matter what the experts say.

I have seen many of my clients go from overweight, pasty, unhealthy people to trim, fit, and energetic individuals. In almost every case, these people tell me, with some amazement: "You know, I don't even *want* those foods anymore." These men and women are living proof that you don't have to be held hostage by impulses that were programmed millions of years ago to protect the body from threats that no longer exist. Instead you can use your understanding of these preferences to help your body thrive in the modern world—and achieve the healthy thin state you have always desired.

PART TWO

SIX STEPS
TO FOOD CONTROL

STEP ONE
KNOW YOUR EATING PRINT

Those who fail to remember the past
are condemned to repeat it.
GEORGE SANTAYANA

If you've ever been to a physician's office, you have probably gone through the sometimes annoying experience of filling out a medical history form, checking off answers to dozens of questions about your past health problems and family history. The fact is, no doctor can make an accurate diagnosis without a thorough understanding of the entire mosaic of the patient's experience.

As with any health care procedure, any weight-loss plan has to be based on an understanding of the many factors that led to your weight problem. Therefore, the first and foremost strategy of weight loss can be summarized in four words: *Learn from your history!*

Pattern Theory

Very early in my career, I became aware of a critical similarity among almost all of my clients. Although they often had very different backgrounds and food preferences, every client who had lost weight and gained it back had done so with the *very same types of food,* in the *very same places,* at the *very same times* of the day, week, and year that had caused them to gain weight in the first place. Clients who were heavy in their midsixties were eating the very same foods that had made them heavy when they were in their thirties and forties. No matter how many times they had tried to lose weight, the overall pattern of their eating behavior—and attitudes toward food—remained the same. And whenever they went back to that pattern, the weight came back.

No matter what your age, ethnic background, religion, or nationality, your weight problem is the result of a combination of biological, psychological, behavioral, and emotional elements that work together to determine your food choices. If you want to change your weight, you need to recognize and change your pattern. And that requires a thorough understanding of your Eating Print, the fingerprint of Food Control Training.

Your Eating Print

Somewhere in the files of the hospital where you were born, there is a sheet of paper bearing your most unique and identifiable characteristic—your fingerprints, which will remain the same throughout your life. Your Eating Print is much the same but is made of the what, how, when, and why of your eating history. It is the sum total of the foods, behaviors, situations, and moods that prompt you to lose control of food in your life. These *trigger foods, trigger behaviors, trigger situations,* and *trigger emotions* never truly leave you. You may diet, you may fast, but ultimately you will return to the pattern of your Eating Print—unless you learn to permanently avoid and control these triggers.

The mouth does not exist in a vacuum. Eating is affected by many subtle (and not-so-subtle) biological, social, cultural, psychological, and situational influences. A person who has no trouble at all eating a scoop of ice cream in a restaurant may eat an entire pint in the privacy of his own kitchen. A woman who has little interest in sweets or peanut butter most of the month may go through an entire bag of Reese's Pieces the day before her period. Food choices change in reaction to many different cues. What sets you off on an eating spree may have no effect at all on your best friend.

There is a probability attached to each food you eat. Some have a high probability that you will lose control, some a low one. A particular food may trigger your appetite to such a degree that even when you try to control the amount you eat, you fail. Or it may be a food that you always turn to in times of stress. Or it may even be a *type* of food (like finger foods) that, once you start, you feel compelled to keep eating regardless of whether you are hungry or even like it.

You undoubtedly already know the foods you like and are inclined to overindulge in. You may even recognize some of the behaviors and situations that prompt you to overeat. What you need to do is put it all together to see the probabilities of and overall *pattern* to your behavior. Your Eating Print is the mirror in which you can see your eating history. Look fearlessly into this mirror, and you will see the foods, behaviors, situations, and moods that have been your downfall in the past. More importantly, if you learn from what you see you will be able to overcome those pitfalls and make it to a comfortable, lasting thin.

In Food Control Training, prevention *is* the cure, and your Eating Print is the "prescription." It will shape every aspect of your weight loss and weight maintenance—from choosing a specific diet plan to choosing a specific food.

THERE CAN BE NO MODERATION, THERE MUST BE ELIMINATION ✧

Trigger Foods:
Why You Can't Have Just One

There's a popular potato chip commercial that offers up the dare "Betcha can't eat just one!" It's a good bet. I have dozens of clients who have said, "Whenever I start on potato chips [or peanuts, or cookies . . .] I can't stop until the bag is empty!" Trigger foods are the ones that you can't "have just one" of—once you've started, you won't stop until the supply runs out. They are the foods that prompt chain eating, and they can be just as difficult to kick as chain smoking.

Perhaps you think that all foods are your trigger foods. Many of my clients thought so. They believed that when they started eating they were unable to stop, no matter what the food. But most people with food control problems are actually susceptible to a relatively small number of very specific foods, usually pretty unhealthy ones.

Let's face it, you didn't gain weight by eating fresh vegetables or shrimp. It takes a lot of asparagus and flounder to make a person fat! No, you've probably gained weight on the high-sugar, high-fat, high-starch "treats" that culture and biology tell us are good, the foods that cause more illness and death in our society (in the form of hypertension, heart disease, diabetes, and various cancers) than any virus. Indeed, I believe *the snack food revolution—the vast proliferation of junk foods (whether they be fat or nonfat) that has overtaken our supermarket shelves in the past twenty-five years—is directly responsible for our nation's rise in obesity.* And this tendency has been aggravated by societal developments like increasing time pressure and a tendency to skip meals and to fill up on snacks.

Most people can easily identify their trigger foods. If you

aren't sure of yours, start by making a list of all your favorite foods. Include any and all types of food, from soup
to nuts—and, of course, junk food.

Once you have your list, read it carefully. Do you notice
a pattern? Do any of the foods belong to a specific food cat-
egory? Are they:

- Sweet foods (candy, cookies, cakes)?
- Foods with a specific texture and mouth feel (i.e.,
  crunchy foods like potato chips, creamy foods like ice
  cream)?
- Finger foods?
- Salty foods (potato chips, pretzels, nacho chips, and so
  on)?
- All of the above?

Rewrite the list, with the similar foods grouped together.
Now subject each item to the Control Test, nine simple
questions that can tell you if you have a consistent history
of abusing a particular food.

THE CONTROL TEST
1. Have you told yourself, "I'll just have one" or "just a
   little" and found it impossible to stick with this commitment?
2. Have you ever tried to give it up entirely and been unable to stay away?
3. When you see this food, do you crave it?
4. Do you eat it even when you're not really hungry?
5. Do you choose this food over other foods that might
   be available?
6. Have you ever eaten it instead of a meal?
7. Do you always eat it in certain situations (e.g., bread

from the bread basket at restaurants, peanuts at the bar, hors d'oeuvres at cocktail parties)?

8. When you dieted in the past did you give it up?
9. When you gained back the weight, were you eating it again?

If your answer to these questions—particularly the last two—is yes, then you have identified a trigger food, a food that has sabotaged your previous attempts to lose weight, a food that has made you fat, and—more than likely—a food you think you love and cannot live without.

Make a final list of all the foods that you've identified as triggers. Study it. Memorize it. See these foods for what they are.

Not treats . . .

Not goodies . . .

Not rewards . . .

Not comfort . . .

Enemies! Enemies that have crept into your life and made you fat. Enemies in an ongoing battle for control of your weight, your health, and your life.

Put next to that list a picture of yourself at your highest weight so you don't forget what these foods have done to you. They haven't done you any favors. They have not made you happy. They have not improved your quality of life. All they have done is add pounds to your weight, taken years off your life, and eroded your sense of self-worth and self-esteem. Any food that you cannot control is controlling you. Don't spend another second of your life hating yourself. Turn your wrath on these foods. They are jailers that have imprisoned you in a lifetime of weight problems.

You must ask yourself, what is the true cost of eating this food for my weight, my control, and my health? These foods are not free. They have a cost. And just as you don't walk into a store and pick out clothes without stopping to check the price tag, you shouldn't walk blindly and carelessly when shopping for food. No food is really free. Some foods, like leafy green vegetables or fruits, give us a bonus when we eat them; others have a very high markup because we end up having to wear them. That is why we should stop allowing our food preferences to be taste bud driven; they must be cost driven.

Trigger foods are a double risk to men and women with weight problems: They are a source of unwanted (and often nonnutritive) calories, and they prompt further losses of control. One slip with a bag of Oreos can be enough to make some people feel they've blown it completely, prompting a general collapse of control of their eating. They may start to skip meals and pick their way through the day. A client who slipped and ate a large bag of pretzels during his lunch hour and followed it with a high-fat dinner and an incredibly rich dessert later told me, "I figured, what the hell, I blew the day anyway!" Like dominoes, once the first bit of control goes, the others soon follow.

Some people call this phenomenon "food addiction" because it is so similar to other addictive processes. There is no question that many foods have dramatic effects on hormone levels and even on the chemistry of the brain itself. But even if we never find a clear psychological cause, the loss of control that is prompted by trigger foods perfectly matches the behavioral consequences of addiction. Like drugs, trigger foods have a destructive effect on your behavior, causing you to lose control despite your determination not to. Whatever the case, one thing is certain: *You don't have to be crazy to be crazy about a cookie!*

Fortunately, very few people succumb to *all* of their trigger foods *all* the time. In fact, most people have very specific susceptibilities to their trigger foods—susceptibilities that are linked to certain behaviors, situations, and moods.

But when you really can't control a specific trigger food, you can't have it both ways. Thin is not free—there is a price, and it may be the elimination of some of your trigger foods from your diet. Only you can decide what is most important to you. Are you willing to trade off one or more of your old "goodies" to reach the thin you've always desired? Are you willing to accept a few limitations in exchange for the freedom of good health?

The Great Lie

Perhaps the greatest threat to maintaining control over trigger foods is the phrase that I call the Great Lie of Dieting: "I'll just have a little!" Every time you fall for the Great Lie you set off on a slippery slope that is ruled by the F/Q Principle of Food Control: Simply, whenever you go back to a trigger food, first the *frequency* increases and then the *quantity* follows suit. It is a slow and insidious process that all too often leads well-meaning and highly motivated people back to the very same foods that made them heavy in the first place. Remember, most people gain back their weight over twelve to eighteen months, not twelve to eighteen days. It's the slow pace of weight gain that prompts the subtle erosion of your resolve.

If you've ever fallen victim to the Great Lie, at first you may have seemed to be getting away with it. You indulged in just a taste of your trigger, without any further harm done . . . that time. But that first "safe" taste gave you a false sense of security. If it worked once, why not twice? And three times? Gradually, the frequency increased. Then the *Q* part of the equation kicked in, and the quantity went up. You started with one or two Oreos, and a few weeks or months later you noticed you were eating more and more. Soon you weren't satisfied until you'd eaten almost an entire bag. Then it went beyond Oreos as you started purchasing ice cream as well, or Doritos, or licorice. . . . Before you knew it, you were back where you started—fat and discouraged.

Don't be too hard on yourself. Logically, an intelligent, motivated person should be able to taste an old problem food and then stop at a little. But reality and logic are rarely in agreement. You can't control a trigger food with logic alone. Taste buds have a memory and power all their own. Once they get a taste of a trigger food, the physiological re-action isn't "Delicious. Thank you, that was enough." It's "Quick! Get me some more!" That small taste triggers a de-sire for more.

When it comes to trigger foods, good intentions simply don't work. Like the road to hell, the road to fat is paved with good intentions. So don't fool yourself with talk of "just a little" or "just this once" because once taste buds are activated, good intentions are all too often swept aside.

The only way to avoid the slippery slope of the F/Q Prin-ciple is to steer clear of the Great Lie. The next time you are tempted to try "just a little" of one of your trigger foods, use the power sentence that has helped thousands of my clients to deflate the Great Lie. Take a deep breath, turn your eyes and your thinking on that trigger food, and tell yourself: *"I don't take the first little taste, I don't begin. I don't have any problem!"*

Some people may think it's easier said than done, but that is not really accurate. When I began this book and asked my clients which of our strategies helped them the most in our work, ideas that helped turn the tide for them against a lifetime of failure with weight control, I was amazed that the overwhelming majority told me, "I don't begin, I don't have any problem."

In the area of trigger foods there can be no equivocation. If a specific food or type of food threatens the quality of your life, that food has to go. If you are absolutely unable to eat it in moderation at any time in your life, then you should not eat it at all. After all, no one who lost and then regained weight ever said, "I think I'll start eating again so I can get fat." No, they all truly believed they could handle their old problem foods, that they could stop at just a little. If 95 percent of dieters (yourself included, perhaps) have been proven wrong, do you really think you can beat the odds? Look in the mirror of your Eating Print and learn from what you see. The lessons can save much more than your figure.

Control is just like a muscle—the more you exercise it by saying "No, thank you," the stronger you become and the easier it becomes to say "No, thank you" in the future.

Trigger Behaviors:
Are Your Fingers Making You Fat?

Have you ever found yourself standing in front of the refrigerator, picking away, and not quite knowing why you were there? Or have you settled in to watch a baseball game, bag of potato chips at your side, and twenty minutes later wondered where they all went? Or have you sat down at the bar and realized that you've finished the bowl of peanuts before you finished your drink?

If you have, welcome to the world of trigger behaviors— the habitual and often almost unconscious behavioral patterns that lead to the repeated abuse of the trigger foods that make you fat. These are the behaviors that prompt you to eat the wrong foods, in the wrong amounts, at the wrong times.

Trigger behaviors can be hard to pin down, since so

many of them are unconscious. The calories are popped into your mouth by the thousands and never register on your mind (although they certainly register on your hips!).

To identify your problem eating behaviors, take the following quiz. The more you understand your trigger behaviors, the more you will be able to control them.

First, grade each statement on a scale of 1 to 5, according to how well it describes your behavior. If it's true of you almost all of the time, give it a 5. If it's something you hardly ever do, score it 1. If it is something you never do, give yourself 0 points for that statement.

PROBLEM EATING BEHAVIORS

1. At parties, I spend a lot of time at the snack table. ___
2. Once I start snacking on hors d'oeuvres, I can't stop. ___
3. I particularly like foods I can eat with my fingers. ___
4. I open the refrigerator door whenever I go into the kitchen. ___
5. I eat while standing up (i.e., at the counter in the kitchen). ___
6. I get "the munchies" when I am bored. ___
7. I believe it is wasteful not to finish everything on my plate or to throw food away. ___
8. Popcorn or candy is a "must" at the movies, even if I've just eaten a meal. ___
9. I have eaten popcorn at the movies instead of a regular meal. ___
10. When baking cookies, I find myself picking at the batter before it goes in the oven. ___

11. If I can't finish a meal at a restaurant, I always get a doggy bag.   —

12. I rarely sit down to a regular meal.   —

13. I tend to eat while I cook, so I'm usually not hungry when the meal is ready to serve.   —

14. At buffets, I like to try a little bit of everything.   —

15. I like easy-to-eat foods like pizza, hot dogs, and burgers.   —

16. I like to have something to snack on while watching TV or reading.   —

17. At restaurants, I can never resist the bread basket.   —

18. The first thing I do when I get home from work is grab a snack to tide me over until dinner.   —

19. I don't eat breakfast.   —

20. At buffets, I like to get my money's worth and go back for second helpings.   —

21. I don't have time for lunch. I just grab a little something in the afternoon.   —

22. I eat while talking on the phone.   —

23. I forget to eat (or don't have time to eat) until the end of the day.   —

24. There are rarely leftovers from meals I eat at home.   —

25. I like to snack after dinner and before going to bed.   —

26. I always seem to go for junk food snacks in the late afternoon (around 3:00 P.M. to 6:00 P.M.).   —

27. I often eat the leftovers while cleaning up after a party in my home.   —

28. I often find myself eating foods that I bought or was saving for company or other family members.   —

Now it's time to determine just what kind of eater you are. Get ready to do a little math. Add the scores for the numbered questions in each of the following columns.

PICKER	PROWLER	FINISHER
1 ____	1 ____	7 ____
2 ____	3 ____	11 ____
3 ____	4 ____	20 ____
4 ____	5 ____	24 ____
5 ____	6 ____	27 ____
8 ____	9 ____	
10 ____	10 ____	TOTAL ____
13 ____	12 ____	Low = below 8.
14 ____	13 ____	Average = 8–12.
16 ____	14 ____	High = above 12.
17 ____	15 ____	
22 ____	17 ____	HOARDER
26 ____	26 ____	18 ____
27 ____		19 ____
28 ____		21 ____
		23 ____
		25 ____

TOTAL ____	TOTAL ____	TOTAL ____
Low = below 20.	Low = below 20.	Low = below 10.
Average = 20–36.	Average = 20–36.	Average = 10–15.
High = above 36.	High = above 36.	High = above 15.

◇ YOU CAN'T EAT IT ALL AND STILL BE THIN ◇ HAPPY OR SAD, RICH OR

If you scored high on the Picker scale, welcome to the club! Ninety-nine percent of my clients are Pickers, people who love finger foods of any kind and who can go through thousands of calories within minutes. Finger foods are the Picker's worst enemy, which is why I say that more people have gained weight with their *fingers* than with their *mouths*. If you are a Picker, for you the essence of weight control is finger control! More people have gained weight from what they eat before, after, and in between meals than from what they consume at the meal itself.

If you're a Picker, there are several simple tricks that you can use to break yourself of the "fat through the fingers" habit.

- Never eat while standing up. If you're standing, you're not paying attention, and if you're not paying attention to your eating, you're not in control.
- No eating while cooking. There's a big difference between taste testing and eating half the muffins as they come out of the oven.
- No eating while on the phone. For one thing, it's rude. For another, it epitomizes uncontrolled and unconscious eating.
- Don't eat with your hands. If it's a finger food, it's a threat, so steer clear of foods that don't require the use of utensils.
- Use your nondominant hand. This is a surprisingly effective and simple trick that works well at any party where finger foods are a fixture. Keep your drink in your dominant hand, so that if you *do* reach for a snack, you'll have to think about it a bit more than usual. You'll be amazed at how difficult it can be to get

a dip-laden chip to your mouth when you're doing it with your nondominant hand.

- Stay out of the kitchen. As often as you can, that is. Try to keep the room reserved for cooking and eating *meals*. Otherwise, stay away. Don't go through your bills at the kitchen table or use the phone there—you're likely to start noshing. If you watch TV late at night, do it in your bedroom or another room away from the refrigerator. And turn out the kitchen light after dinner; a dark room may deflect thoughts of a midnight snack.

- Beware the bread basket. Almost all restaurants offer up some form of bread, muffins, or other finger food before you have even ordered. These baskets of temptation can be lethal to Pickers. Either ask that it be removed, ask your companions to keep the bread basket on their side of the table, or turn over your bread plate.

If you *have* to have some kind of snack, live by this axiom: "Nothing in the fingers except shrimp (at parties), vegetables, allowed fruit, or a diet beverage." In other words, pickles are okay, corn chips aren't!

If you are a Prowler you have a lot in common with Pickers—with one crucial difference. Pickers will eat a lot between meals, but they will eat meals. Prowlers rarely sit down to three real meals a day. They snack their way through the day, grabbing a roll here, a sandwich there, but hardly ever actually sitting down to a complete meal. Prowlers rely on quick, easy foods that often have many calories and few nutrients. If you're a Prowler, people around you may think you never eat, since you never take the time to have breakfast, lunch, and dinner. But if you took an accurate inventory of how much you consume during the average day, you'd probably be shocked at how many calories you take in.

Most of the tricks that work for Pickers will work equally with Prowlers, with a few crucial additions:

- Never skip a meal. Prowlers are always saying they don't have time to eat, even though they are basically eating all the time. Make time in your day for real meals, not snacks on the run, and don't skip any.

- Always sit down while eating. A meal isn't a meal if it's eaten on the run, or at a counter, or in the car on the way to work. Prowlers need to establish a healthy, consistent meal pattern, and sitting down to eat can help that.

- Focus on your meals. Don't eat while watching television, or reading a book, or trying to finish that report that was due last week. Prowlers tend to eat without awareness, so when you do eat, enjoy it! Pay attention to what, where, and when you are eating.

- Beware the ten-minute problem. Prowlers are most in their element in the first few moments after they arrive home (or at a party or restaurant). It is during those first ten minutes—before the meal has been served—that you are most likely to nosh on whatever food is available. So be careful! Hold out till your scheduled meal.

Finishers are members of the "clean plate club." If you scored high on this scale, your grandmother might be pleased, but your waistline isn't. You've learned too well the lessons of your childhood: "It's wrong to waste food." "There are starving people in the world." "Always get what you pay for."

Conquering the Finisher habit often means making some fairly major changes in your beliefs and attitudes about food, but you can get a good head start by observing two primary precautions:

- Don't overload your plate. If it's on your plate, you are going to feel obligated to eat it.
- Eat more slowly. Give yourself at least twenty minutes to eat your meals so your body has a chance to satiate itself and you have a chance to enjoy them.

Hoarders, unlike Prowlers and Pickers, eat on the *layaway plan*. They tend to ignore food during the day when they are running around dealing with the work of their daily life. They hoard their hunger until the evening, when work is done and they are at home or at a restaurant. Then, ravenous, they finally eat all the calories they should have had earlier in the day. Since by then they are extremely hungry, they make poor food choices and continue eating well into the night hours— when their bodies are least able to burn the calories and most likely to store them as fat. Like Prowlers, Hoarders often seem to be people who "never eat" because they hardly ever sit down to a meal with other people. In general, Hoarders benefit from following the same precautions as Prowlers—they are best off if they actually schedule their meals and then stick to that schedule. This prevents the ravenous hunger that so often hits them at the end of the day.

Trigger behaviors, like every other aspect of eating, rarely occur in a vacuum. Many are very situation-specific. An inveterate Picker, for example, is in his element at a cocktail party, where trays of seductive treats pass by his fingers at all times. In this situation, a world-class Picker can consume several thousand calories without even realizing he's eating. So knowing *when* you are triggered to eat is just as important as knowing *what* triggers you and *how* you do it.

Trigger Situations: It's Not What You Eat But Where and When You Eat It

No one eats *all* the time. You, like everyone else on the planet, have moments when you eat without thinking and moments when you don't think about eating. Knowing which moments are trigger situations and which are not can make all the difference.

Trigger situations, along with trigger behaviors and trigger foods, form the Bermuda Triangle of dieting—a region where dieters easily lose their way. Trigger situations prompt you to eat even when you are not hungry. They put you on automatic pilot, so that food reaches your mouth almost without your being aware of it.

The most common situational triggers are those involved with preparing and sharing food—particularly social situations: parties with generous trays of hors d'oeuvres, attending a buffet luncheon and having seconds or thirds "because it's free," going out to dinner with friends and going through three bread baskets and several shared appetizers before the entrées even arrive. All of these situations can elicit unconscious and uncontrolled eating, particularly if the foods involved are among your triggers.

Over the years, I have found that people who are susceptible to trigger situations can be grouped into two categories, *Cooks* and *Noncooks*. To determine which group you fall into, take the following quiz. Grade each statement according to how well it describes your behavior. If it's true of you almost all of the time, give it a 5. If it's something you hardly ever do, give it a 1. If it is something you never do, give yourself 0 points for that statement.

PROBLEM EATING SITUATIONS

1. At the movies, I always buy popcorn or a snack.   —
2. I eat more on the weekends than I do during the week.   —
3. I like to have something to munch on while watching TV.   —
4. I eat out in restaurants more often than I do at home.   —
5. When cleaning up after a party, I snack on the leftovers.   —
6. I find it hard to eat sensibly at friends' houses or in restaurants.   —
7. My refrigerator and cupboard are filled with snack foods and easy-to-prepare foods.   —
8. I send out for food more often than I cook.   —
9. I like to cook and make most of my own meals.   —
10. I eat more at home than I do in restaurants or at parties.   —
11. On the weekends or my days off, I am rarely at home.   —
12. I eat while talking on the phone.   —
13. My refrigerator and cupboard are practically empty, but I have a lot of take-out menus.   —
14. I like to spend my weekends or days off at home, puttering around the house or relaxing.   —

MORE PEOPLE HAVE GAINED WEIGHT FROM EATING STANDING UP

15. I like easy-to-eat foods like pizza, hot dogs, and burgers. ___
16. At restaurants, I'm often full before the entrée arrives because the rolls in the bread basket are so good. ___
17. The first thing I do when I get home from work is to grab a snack to tide me over until dinner. ___
18. I like to snack after dinner and before going to bed. ___

COOK		NONCOOK	
2	___	1	___
3	___	4	___
5	___	6	___
7	___	7	___
9	___	8	___
10	___	11	___
12	___	13	___
14	___	15	___
17	___	16	___
18	___		

TOTAL ___
Low = below 20.
Average = 20–30.
High = above 30.

TOTAL ___
Low = below 18.
Average = 18–27.
High = above 27.

Cooks, as you might guess, tend to do most of their overeating at home where foods are convenient, witnesses few, and time available. Noncooks, on the other hand, tend to get their food outside the home at parties, in restaurants, or from fast-food outlets. Although Noncooks do sometimes eat in their homes, they rarely have much food on hand and generally have to send out for it. Noncooks may like food, but they're hardly ever Cooks.

This is not to say that all Cooks eat perfectly in public or that all Noncooks are safe in their own kitchens. There are certain times of the day and week that are triggers for almost everyone, anywhere. For example:

- The first quarter hour after getting home from work is particularly dangerous, since you are often hungry and fatigued and are most likely to pick at trigger foods during this time.
- Women who work in the home are often at high risk in the late afternoon—between the hours of 3:00 P.M. and 6:00 P.M.
- Watching TV
- And almost everyone seems to have more problems with their appetite on lazy weekend afternoons while lounging around the house. Boredom or just having unstructured free time on your hands can encourage nonstop noshing and the feeling of being hungry.

In general, the problem with trigger situations is not the situations themselves, it's your *reaction* to them. Most of us react to our trigger situations like well-rehearsed actors in a long-running play. We pick up our "cue"—be it a pretzel, a stuffed mushroom, or a miniature cream puff—without thought. We're like Pavlov's dogs: The bell rings (or the tray comes out) and we're off and eating!

It isn't mere chance that the most potent trigger situations are often the most social and festive. All of us have deep psychological and emotional links to food, and this fact is responsible for the next class of triggers, trigger emotions.

Trigger Emotions:
Can Calories Make You Happy?

Sometimes eating or feeling hungry is not about food. People often eat when they are lonely, frustrated, sad, or angry, choosing foods in response to emotional rather than physical needs.

Of course, not everyone eats because of emotional disturbances in their lives. Food is more comforting to some people than it is to others. But it is a fact that for many people emotional eating is a big part of their weight problem. Instead of coping with painful or difficult emotions, they use food as a panacea. They become Food Therapists. When the going gets tough, they stuff.

Food *can* be very comforting, it's true. But for Food Therapists, food is the only comfort. They have developed a one-word response to any and all problems: "Eat!"

To determine if—or how much—you are a Food Therapist, rate each statement on a scale of 1 to 5. A rating of 1 means the statement is rarely true of you, a rating of 5 means it is almost always true. If you completely disagree with the statement, the score is 0.

DO YOU USE FOOD AS THERAPY?

1. There is no problem that can't be solved with chocolate. ___
2. I like to treat myself to a nice dinner (or some other food treat) to celebrate accomplishments or a job well done. ___
3. On previous diets, I've sometimes cheated because I just felt I deserved a little treat. ___

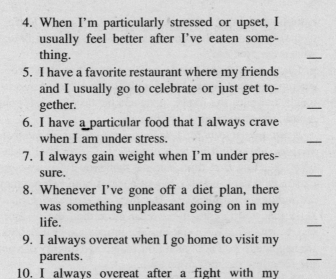

4. When I'm particularly stressed or upset, I usually feel better after I've eaten something. ___

5. I have a favorite restaurant where my friends and I usually go to celebrate or just get together. ___

6. I have a particular food that I always crave when I am under stress. ___

7. I always gain weight when I'm under pressure. ___

8. Whenever I've gone off a diet plan, there was something unpleasant going on in my life. ___

9. I always overeat when I go home to visit my parents. ___

10. I always overeat after a fight with my boyfriend/girlfriend/husband/wife. ___

TOTAL ___

If you scored 21 or less, you're doing pretty well—you may occasionally turn to food for solace, but you're basically an unemployed Food Therapist. If you scored 22 to 36, you are employed as a Food Therapist on a part-time basis. But if you scored 37 or more, you are one of the legions of people who turn to food first and foremost to solve (or at least temporarily relieve) your distress.

To be fair, it's perfectly natural to turn to food for comfort on occasion. I don't know anyone who isn't a Food Therapist at least once in a while—if only when having a bowl of hot chicken soup on a gray rainy day.

Perhaps because of this, some of my clients have asked whether it really matters if they use food as a remedy for emotional stress. "After all," they say, "if I'm not terribly overweight and if the food actually makes me feel better, what's the problem?"

These people are missing the point. Ultimately, Food Therapy doesn't work. You may feel better for a few moments, but once the food is gone and the taste has left your mouth, the original problem remains.

If you turn to food for solace, you are confusing immediate pleasure with long-term happiness. The alcohol addict who takes that first drink and the dangerously overweight person who eats an entire bag of cookies both believe they are indulging in pleasures. But they are *destructive pleasures* that will eventually cost far more than the pleasure was worth. Whenever you mistake immediate gratification for happiness, you are risking the length and quality of your life for a few seconds of pleasure.

This is the real world. This is not Disneyland. There will always be stresses and tension in your life. If you respond with only one word—*eat!*—then you have tied your weight to what's going on around you instead of what is right for your body and health. When you eat because of someone or some feeling, you are giving that person or feeling *power* over you.

If you are one of the millions of people who eats whenever someone annoys or hurts you, *stop!* Don't let that person win twice—first by hurting you, then by making you fat. Refuse to let that person be so powerful in your life. Take back the power and use it against destructive eating, not against yourself. Don't cheat yourself out of a thin (and healthy) future.

Calories cannot make you happy. Food cannot resolve stressful situations. Food will not help you cope. Food will not teach you new skills to deal with stress. It will not repair your relationships. Instead, it will block your development and make you dependent on an external substance to cope. As long as your eating is tied to your emotions, you will never achieve a stable weight. Your weight will change as often as your emotions do. And any diet—no matter how sound—will be as futile as trying to build a castle in the sand. It will be swept away with the next wave of emotion.

Emotional eating turns you into an emotional cheapskate; you don't give yourself enough credit for what you can handle. Instead of telling yourself that you "can deal with these feelings" and "feelings pass," you start believing that you "just can't deal" with your feelings without food in your hand.

You deserve better than that and you can have it. Just as you can become more physically fit through exercise and healthy living, you can become more psychologically fit. You can learn the difference between coping and consumption, between instant gratification and happiness. You can learn to manage your weight by learning to manage your *life*—without turning to food. After all, if you control an empire but feel out of control with your own body, how can you truly enjoy your successes?

You've got to recognize this when you turn to food and consciously remind yourself that food is not going to solve the problem or relieve the feeling. When you find yourself reaching for your particular "food tranquilizer," stop! Think about not just what it tastes like but what it is going to do to you. Ask yourself:

- What kind of "reward" makes you miserable five minutes later?
- What kind of "treat" makes you throw out the clothes you once loved?

- What kind of "cure" ruins your looks, your health, and your self-esteem?

You can use your knowledge of your Eating Print to become a good *self-therapist,* to spot the trouble situations and behaviors before they occur and take steps to protect yourself. And by understanding your Eating Print, you can better remind yourself of what food did and did not do for you in the past. Namely, it did make you fat and it did not make you happy.

Putting It Together

Now that you have charted out the specifics of your Eating Print, take a moment to review what you have learned. What food or foods always seem to prompt you to uncontrolled eating? In what situations? In what moods? Does your favorite food serve as a trigger only when you actually have it in the house? Do you lose control of it only when you are angry or stressed? Use your Eating Print to shed light on the overall pattern of your eating history. More than likely, you will see that you are not out of control with *food* in general, but only with a few *select foods,* in very specific situations.

Your Eating Print is more than a window onto your past, it is also a crystal ball to your future. The Eating Print is the law of gravity of weight control—irresistible and incontrovertible. If your Eating Print shows that you consistently abused a food in the past, you can know with certainty that you will abuse it in the future.

For many of my clients, uncovering the Eating Print is the most liberating and reassuring moment of Food Control Training. Cooks who thought they were hopeless binge eaters discovered that they were really at risk in only one area—the kitchen of their own homes. Pickers who thought they needed some ascetic program of weight control discovered that what they really needed was finger control. And Hoarders who believed they could never control the ravenous hunger that hit them at the end of the day learned that all they really needed was a regular eating schedule.

For the first time, these men and women are able to see their weight problem for what it is—*not a mountain to climb, but a few specific patterns to master.* Suddenly, the prospect of losing weight does not seem so daunting, so hopeless. It is truly attainable. You can see that, too. The Eating Print will help you see further and more clearly than you've been able to before, beyond what is on your plate or counter, beyond the end of your nose to the true value of your life.

STEP TWO
DEFINE YOUR PERSONAL THIN

One can never be too thin or too rich.
THE DUCHESS OF WINDSOR

Do you want to know the secret to losing as much weight as you want? It's simple:

GET REAL!

Perhaps no one has ever told you this basic truth. Well, that's it. Before you can *get thin,* you have to get real about your weight, get real about your life, and get real about the goals you set for yourself.

First, let's make it clear what thin is *not.* Thin is not an arbitrary number on a scale. It's not the cover of *Cosmopolitan* or *GQ.* It is not the model of the moment or the latest celebrity fitness adviser.

Thin is personal. Thin is unique. Thin is the weight that improves your health, appearance, and overall quality of life. It is the weight that allows you to walk up a flight of stairs—briskly—but doesn't require utter starvation to get there. It is the weight that looks and feels great on you and that everybody will notice. Thin is the weight that you will be able to achieve—and maintain—within the realities of your day-to-day life.

Losing weight is a private, personal matter. Yet many people turn to some arbitrary weight table or chart to deter-

---

❖ YOU'VE COME TOO FAR IN LIFE TO TAKE ORDERS FROM A COOKIE! ❖

mine their "ideal" weight as if there's one magic number that each person should (or should not) weigh. But there isn't. In the real world, only one person knows the weight that will work for you—*you*.

More than likely, when you've set goals for yourself in the past, you've made them too difficult. Most people I've known who were seeking to lose weight didn't need to lose nearly as much as they thought. That's true for almost everyone, and I guarantee that's true for you, too—whether you weigh 150 or 350.

Yes, you want to be leaner, but you also want to *stay* at that lean weight. So be healthy and realistic in setting your goals.

That's what the winners have done, and that's why the winners of weight control come in all different shapes and sizes. And that's why figuring out a *realistic* weight goal is an important strategy for achieving a comfortable—and lasting—thin.

Taking the First Step

Every year, dieters the world over give up on losing weight because they set unattainable goals for themselves. If you are one of these people, it is time for you to take a good hard look at yourself, your history, and your life and start thinking in terms of your *tolerable* or *winnable* weight rather than some mythic ideal. If you have a specific weight goal in mind and if you were ever at this goal weight, ask yourself the following questions:

- How old were you at the time?
- How long did you stay at this weight?
- How much were you exercising?
- What were you eating?

If you were only at this weight for a short time and if your life was substantially different from the one you live now, reconsider your goal. If you're a man who used to play varsity football and now cannot even find time for a weekend pickup game in the park or if you're a woman who has been on the Pill or who has been pregnant since the time you were at your goal weight, it is definitely time to redefine your target.

Sometimes the weight you can maintain is the "ideal weight" of the tables and charts. Sometimes it isn't. Instead of focusing on that "perfect" number on your scale, start thinking in terms of range—a range of numbers that would provide an acceptable and achievable span for your weight. Quick-loss diets that get you down to some fairy-tale weight are like a hundred-yard dash, exhilarating but short-lived. *Living* thin is for the long run—a journey that takes you across many different terrains at different speeds and will give you a prolonged sense of accomplishment. Food Control Training is designed to turn out runners who endure and triumph rather than falter after the first mile.

Facing the Mirror

First, take a good look at yourself in a full-length mirror. Ideally, look at yourself in the nude—after you've showered or just before you dress. Spend some time at it. Really look at your body. Note where you tend to accumulate fat. Is it around your waist? Your thighs? Your back? Your face and neck? Where are your problem spots?

Evaluate just how fit you look. If your arms are full, does the flesh sag or is it firm? If your thighs are heavy, are they dimpled and jiggly or smooth and fairly tight? Can you see any muscle definition in your abdomen, legs, and arms, or are the muscles completely obscured by fat? Take an inventory of the areas that need to be toned and tightened.

Of course, it's almost impossible to look at yourself without comparing yourself to something or someone. Please, for your own sake and sanity, resist the impulse. In fact, try to stick to two basic rules:

1. Forget the Media! If you use the world of entertainment as your guide to an ideal weight, you will only make yourself anxious, depressed, and confused. An ideal is, by definition, "a mental image existing in fancy or imagination only . . . lacking practicality." The images that assault you from movie screens, magazine covers, and billboards have very little to do with good health or the way real people live.

Your goal weight should be just that—*your* weight, not Cindy Crawford's or Sylvester Stallone's, not the weight of any other sex symbol of the moment.

2. Forget the Prom Dress (or Tux)! Too often, dieters look back to some time in their past when they felt particularly slender and beautiful—be it a prom, a wedding day, or a particularly grand vacation—and decide that *that* is the weight they want to reach. It does not matter that they were at that weight twenty-five years ago, or that they ate nothing but iceberg lettuce for six months to get there.

You've probably done it yourself while preparing for a high school reunion, an anniversary party, or a landmark birthday. You looked into the mirror and thought of how much you would like to be back in the shape you were that one glorious summer when you felt young, perfect, and on top of the world. When push comes to shove, however, not many of us really want to turn the clock back. We just wouldn't mind having the body back.

Well, you can't have it. As we age, the body's metabolic efficiency decreases at a rate of about 2 percent per decade. Part of this drop is because of a loss of muscle mass—a factor that can be controlled, at least in part, through regular exercise. But even with exercise, time does have an influence. That's why you need a new vision to strive for—one that sees your body for what it is and can be, not what it once was.

As you look at yourself in that mirror, let go of your old notions of thin and your ideal shape. Simply see your body as it is now, lumps, bumps, cellulite, and all. As you gaze at your body, the parts you love, the parts you hate, or those you haven't really considered in years, imagine your problem areas gradually shrinking. Picture those lumps and bumps becoming smooth lines and contours. Imagine the muscles beneath your fat growing toned and strong. *See yourself, only better.* Fix that image in your mind. Let it take the place of all the other, unrealistic ideals you may have envisioned. And let it be your guide and inspiration as you start on the road to thin.

Choosing a Target

Now that you've given yourself a vision, it's time to set a more concrete target—a specific weight range. In setting this goal, you need to keep in mind another important rule of Food Control Training: *Forget the scale!* You'll need a scale to keep track of your weight, of course, but achieving thin is much more than just losing pounds. Numbers on a scale can be deceiving. Muscle is denser and heavier than fat, so a man who is five feet ten, 195 pounds, and only 12 percent fat will look much thinner than a man who is the same height and weight but 30 percent fat. If you are doing

WHEN YOUR THIN IS TOO THIN

When I say I want you to be thin, I don't mean I want you to be emaciated. I am not using the word *thin* as it has been used (and abused) by a group whom I call the thinnists. The thinnists of our society propagate an unfair standard of beauty for women based on an artificially low weight, which places a terrible burden on them and often leads to eating disorders like anorexia and bulimia. For some, it also makes the word *thin* a feminist issue.

That is not what your Personal Thin is about. I am not advocating the unhealthy cult of thinness that currently plagues our society. Indeed, I have spent at least as much time discouraging my clients from going too low as I have spent encouraging them to lose more weight. But the fact remains that today thin means *healthy*—and you cannot ignore that. As more and more medical research points out, by losing even just a little weight, you reduce your risk for a host of maladies from breast cancer to diabetes to heart disease. Is it antifeminist to encourage women to live a life that will protect them from the ravages of cancer? Is it wrong to encourage *anyone*, man or woman, to take care of his or her body and feel good about him- or herself?

That is what I want the word *thin* to do, and so I advocate a new and healthier use of the word.

things right, no matter how many pounds you lose, you will gain some of them back as added muscle. And that's great, because muscle is metabolically active. The higher your percentage of muscle, the more efficiently you will burn calories.

There is a subtle but consistent loss of muscle mass that comes with each decade of adult life—if you do nothing at all to tone and firm it up, that is. By seeing a truer picture of what your body really looks like, you may find that the best way to counteract the flab factor is not to lose weight so much as gain muscle.

Since weight is such an inaccurate gauge of fitness, we are going to use two other methods to determine your ideal weight range: the Body Mass Index (BMI) and the Body Fat Percentage (BFP).

The Body Mass Index (page 74) is a measure of your body's total mass. The categories—Acceptable, Overweight, and Obese—are based on research concerning the health effects of the various degrees of body mass. People with BMIs in the Acceptable range tend to live longer, with fewer health problems, than those in the higher BMI ranges. So your goal is to keep your body mass within the Acceptable range.

Calculating Your Body Mass Index

To determine your BMI, find your height (in inches) in the right column and your weight (in pounds) in the left column. (Be honest. Don't say you are six feet tall if you are really five-eleven, and don't say 150 pounds when you're really 158.) Using a ruler, draw a straight line between the two points. Your BMI is where the line crosses the middle column.

To determine how much you need to weigh to be in the Acceptable range, keep one end of the ruler on your height and adjust the angle so the ruler crosses the Acceptable portion of the middle column. Draw two more lines—one with your ruler crossing the bottom of the Acceptable column, one at the top.

For example, a woman 5'6" (sixty-six inches) tall who weighs 178 pounds has a BMI of 29—at the high end of the Overweight range. To get to the Acceptable range (a BMI of 19 to 23), she will need to slim down to between 116 and 142 pounds.

The BMI gives you a good measure of your overall mass,

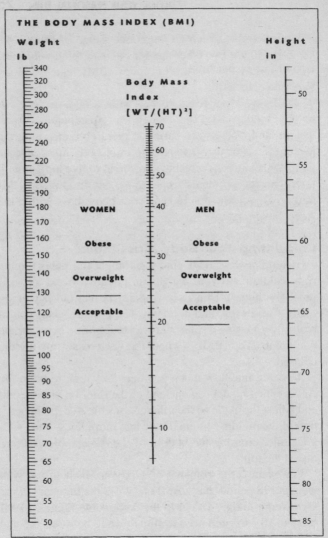

THE BODY MASS INDEX (BMI)

Weight

lb

340
320
300
280
260
240
220
200
190
180
170
160
150
140
130
120
110
100
95
90
85
80
75
70
65
60
55
50

Body Mass Index [WT/(HT)²]

70
60
50
40
30
20
10

WOMEN

Obese

Overweight

Acceptable

MEN

Obese

Overweight

Acceptable

Height

in

50
55
60
65
70
75
80
85

WEIGHT LOSS WILL FOLLOW ◇ IT'S BETTER TO WEAR ITALIAN THAN TO but it does not tell you how much of that mass is fat or lean. For that, we must turn to the Body Fat Percentage and Lean Body Mass (see below).

Calculating Your Body Fat Percentage

First, if you are a woman, measure your hips; if you are a man, measure your waist. (Again, be honest.) Using the tables on pages 77 and 78 find your height in the right column and draw a straight line between your height and your waist or hip girth. Your BFP is where the line crosses the center column.

For example, our five-foot six-inch woman has forty-five-inch hips, so her BFP is 40 percent, meaning that 40 percent of her weight is fat.

The recommended BFP for women is between 16 and 26 percent, with 21 percent a good average for most women. In men, a BFP of 15 percent is considered acceptable, with a range of 12 to 17 percent. Obviously, the woman in our example is carrying an unhealthy percentage of fat. But how many pounds does she need to lose?

Calculating Lean Body Mass

To arrive at a goal weight using the BFP, you need to do some math. The first stage is calculating Lean Body Mass (LBM):

- Multiply your actual weight by the BFP: $178 \times 40\%$ (or .40) = 71.2
- Subtract that result from your actual weight to get your LBM: $178 - 71.2 = 106.8$
- Divide your LBM by .79 (for women) or .85 (for men) to get your goal weight: $106.8 \div .79 = 135.2$

EAT ITALIAN! ❖ I DON'T TAKE THE FIRST LITTLE TASTE, I DON'T BEGIN. I

So, in this example, the woman's ideal weight would be around 135 pounds.

When taken together, the BMI and BFP give you a healthy weight range to strive for. The BMI provides the broad goals—in this case, the high end of the range would be 142 pounds and the low end would be 116. So our 178-pound woman could lose anywhere from thirty-six to sixty-two pounds and still be within a healthy acceptable weight range.

The BFP/LBM helps you hone in even further, to the area on that weight range that will probably be easiest for you to maintain based on your individual body structure. In this case, a BFP/LBM of 135 indicates our sample woman doesn't *have* to get all the way down to 116; she can shoot for the higher end of that range and still end up feeling healthy and looking great.

For the purposes of Food Control Training, there are only two truly guiding principles to deciding your specific target weight: *Stay within your acceptable range* and *strive for the weight you can maintain in real life.*

Tolerable Weight and the Capacity for Change

Your weight is influenced by a variety of factors. Some are changeable, some aren't. There's not much you can do about your genetic code, your age, or your gender. If you are a thirty-seven-year-old woman whose parents were born in Italy, that's where you're going to stay. If you woke up this morning as a forty-five-year-old man whose father is morbidly obese and whose mother has high blood pressure, you'll have the same family history tomorrow. In many ways, your family medical history is like the stars that predict your own medical future.

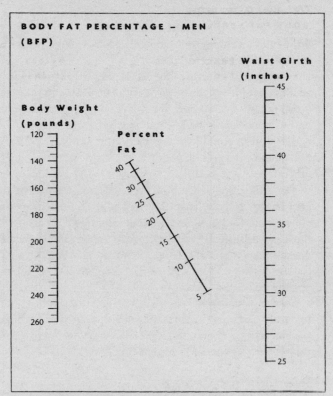

BODY FAT PERCENTAGE – MEN (BFP)

Waist Girth (inches)
- 45
- 40
- 35
- 30
- 25

Body Weight (pounds)
- 120
- 140
- 160
- 180
- 200
- 220
- 240
- 260

Percent Fat
- 40
- 30
- 25
- 20
- 15
- 10
- 5

From *Sensible Fitness*, copyright © 1986 by Jack Wilmore, Ph.D. Published by Leisure Press, a division of Human Kinetics Publishers, Inc.

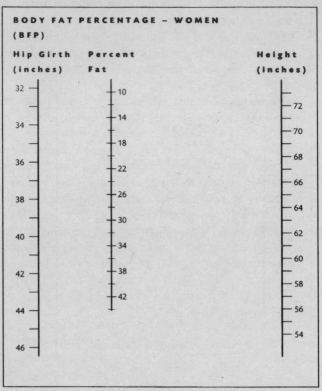

BODY FAT PERCENTAGE — WOMEN (BFP)

Hip Girth (inches)	Percent Fat	Height (inches)
32	10	72
34	14	70
36	18	68
38	22	66
40	26	64
42	30	62
44	34	60
46	38	58
	42	56
		54

From *Sensible Fitness*, copyright © 1986 by Jack Wilmore, Ph.D. Published by Leisure Press, a division of Human Kinetics Publishers, Inc.

This simple fact of life has made some people despair. "My genes are my destiny!" they declare, perhaps pointing to a long line of overweight relatives. "How can I fight them?"

To be perfectly honest, you can't fight your genes. But you can outmaneuver them. Genetics *impels;* it does not *compel.* It's your food choices that ultimately make you heavy, not your genes. Genetics and body structure set the lower limit for your obtainable weight, but you, your food choices, and exercise set the upper limit. For every fixed influence on your weight, there is at least one other factor that you can directly change and control.

Your tolerable weight will largely be determined by how willing you are to make adjustments in the "weight factors" that are under your control. These factors can be broken down into three categories:

- *What* you will eat
- *When* you will eat
- *How* (and how much) you will *move*

"Big deal!" I hear you cry. "I already knew that. What difference is it supposed to make?"

Plenty. Controlling these three relatively simple parts of your behavior can make an enormous difference, not just in your outward appearance, but in the most basic biochemical workings of your body—not to mention improving your overall lifestyle, which is the ultimate determinant of your weight. With a few *permanent* changes in your diet, eating schedule, and activity level, you can completely change the quality—and quantity—of your life.

If you've been on a diet you already know how much of an effect temporary control and restrictions can have. The problem is in making those changes permanent. The fixed factors that influence your weight never go away and tend to become more fat inducing with time. Genes—and the nature of aging—cannot be denied. Men are men, women are women, and time takes its toll on everyone. This is the reality. The person you are now is not the person you were when you were sixteen and is not the person you will be at sixty. Given these facts, how much time and effort are you willing to invest in keeping your weight down?

How to Outmaneuver Your Genes

What you eat and how much you move are the two basic determinants of your Resting Metabolic Rate (RMR). The RMR is a measure of how many calories your body uses to run its basic processes—from growing your toenails to filling your lungs with air to pumping blood through your veins. As you sit reading this book, your body is busily at work with the business of keeping you alive.

The RMR can be very temperamental. It demands a certain base level of calories in order to do its job and if you try to trick it by restricting those calories, the RMR simply goes on a sit-down strike. It burns *less* calories and waits for you to get over this silly diet business. So just as you can't fool your genes, you can't fool your RMR. But you can rev it up.

Your resting metabolic rate has a direct relationship to your working metabolic rate. You can increase the rate at which your body burns calories simply by doing something active every day. With every bout of activity, even if it is just taking the stairs instead of the elevator, you are sending a message to the RMR to speed up. And the more active you are, the more powerful the message. In the book *Genetic Nutrition,* Artemis P. Simopoulos, M.D., Victor Herbert, M.D., J.D., and Beverly Jacobson report that when experimental subjects exercised at six times their resting level, the genetic influences that had seemed to be repressing their RMR simply vanished! In the words of the authors, "one can overcome one's genetic limitations."

Not only that, an average of twenty-one minutes of life would be gained and an average of fifty-three cents in medical and associated costs would be saved for each additional mile walked or run by a sedentary person, according to some estimates.

Clearly, if you want to overcome *your* genetic limitations you are going to have to decide to *move*—and move consistently.

I have a few clients who actually devote most of their lives to molding and perfecting their bodies. They pay thousands of dollars for personal trainers, spend hours at the health club, and eat diets that a Zen monk would find spartan. For them, it's worth it. If you have the time and resources, feel free to pursue that ideal. But remember, there are thousands of winners out there, and they didn't all have access to Heather Locklear's personal trainer and hours upon hours of time to work out. If you are like me (and the majority of my clients), you probably have other priorities.

The point is that it does not take a great deal of time and energy to live healthfully. On the contrary, it's not a matter of spending endless hours, but simply of consistency and staying focused. Eating the right foods doesn't take any more time than eating the wrong foods—it just takes a little planning.

Only you can decide what your tolerable weight is and only you can know when you have reached it. If you can reach—and maintain—the weight you were during some pleasant time in your past, great! If you don't quite make that but get to the acceptable range we discussed, terrific! Even if you "only" succeed at losing half of what you had planned to lose *but keep it off,* bravo!

Every pound you lose and keep off is a move forward on the road to control, self-assurance, and freedom from the tyranny of food. I have worked with thousands of clients— some of whom may have been heavier than you, some of whom may have been thinner—who have taken this road, each at his or her own pace. I can assure you that with each step the path becomes smoother and clearer. In the next chapter, I will show you how to draw the map that will take you further down your own road to thin—whatever that thin may be.

STEP THREE
DITCH DEPRIVATION

*For those given to extremes, abstinence is
easier than moderation.*
JOHN DRYBRED

*There's a considerable difference between
doing without a thing of your own accord,
and being made to do without it.*
ELIZA LESLIE

"I want it—now!"

Did you ever say that as a kid? Most of us did. Unfortunately, when it comes to food, many of us are still saying it. In fact, where food is concerned even the most mature adults often act like children. In fact, we act like brats—Food Brats.

For most people, the idea of permanently saying "no" to a trigger food is completely alien. Suggest it and they suddenly turn into two-year-olds. Digging in their heels, they say, "Give up my french fries (or ice cream, peanuts, cookies, chips . . .)? I can't do that! It's my favorite! I can't live without it."

The fact that their "favorite" has made them fat, unhealthy, and miserable completely escapes them. They are caught in the foodie culture's *deprivation mind-set*, the

mind-set that says restrictions are *bad*—you should be able
to have it all and *still* be thin. Like children who want their
way no matter what, they don't care about the negative consequences of their eating. They have fallen victim to the
Food Brat Syndrome.

Sound familiar? Take a look at your own Eating Print.
How many times have *you* returned to the foods, places, or
behaviors that shot old efforts of weight loss right out of
the water? And how often was it because you felt like you
were being deprived of your favorite "goodies" and
"treats"?

The lesson of the third weight-loss strategy is simple: To
win at weight loss, *ditch the deprivation mind-set!* Ditch
the food-centered beliefs that make you feel deprived. It's
time not just to change your weight, but to change your
thinking about food.

That's what the winners have done. They have learned to
see these foodie beliefs for what they truly are: misprecep-
tions, half-truths, and myths. The myths of deprivation are
based on a denial of reality: They focus on a few minutes'
worth of taste, how it feels in your mouth, and completely
deny the cost. These foods are not free—you have to wear
them for years to come.

If you have fallen under the spell of the deprivationists,
you are in denial. You cannot eat it all and still be thin. This
is not a principle of my program; it is a principle of reality.
And if you have trouble accepting it you are having trouble
with reality, not with Food Control Training.

Only children live their lives believing they can have it
all without any cost. It's time to bring this part of your life
into the adult world. All of life contains adjustments and
trade-offs. In accepting this, you not only establish a frame-
work for a lasting solution to your weight problem, but you

become a more resilient and mature human being. *It's time to stop resenting what you do to keep your body healthy and attractive.* Everything you value in your life—relationships with your life partner and children, your career—has taken work, focus, and endurance. Why should it be any different when it comes to food?

The winners have come to this realization and no longer feel deprived but liberated. In a recent survey of my patients, 84 percent said they felt no deprivation. Without taking this step of growth and maturation, there can be no permanent weight loss, no permanent freedom.

If you've come this far, you are already well on your way to that sense of freedom. You have a realistic idea of the amount of weight you need to lose and you know your Eating Print. You've revealed the mosaic of your history with food. Now you will learn to see that mosaic in the plain light of day, without letting foodie beliefs color your perceptions. You need to explode the deprivation myths that have kept you enslaved to food and free yourself to get on with the business of getting—and living—thin.

Myth 1: Saying "No" to Food Is Saying "Yes" to Deprivation

Deprivation doesn't just happen, it's something that is done to you. The dictionary tells us so. A person who is deprived has been stripped of some "necessity of life or healthful environmental influence by an external person or force." Children living in poverty are deprived. Families trapped in war-torn cities are deprived. Prisoners on starvation rations are deprived. They have no choice, no control over their situation.

By this definition, it is virtually impossible for most middle-class Americans to be truly *deprived* of food. Because the fact is, you can eat *anything* you want, *anytime* you want!

Every diet you have ever tried has proven this point. No one—not me, not your doctor, not even your spouse—can *force* you to avoid a food. Other people can beg, nag, badger, bribe, or even threaten you, but ultimately the decision to eat or not to eat is always yours. No one can take it away from you.

A few years ago, an overweight man at a dinner party told me he had gone off his last diet because he was "tired of feeling punished." The question that immediately came to my mind was, punished by whom? No one was holding a gun to his head. No one was threatening him with divorce or unemployment if he didn't stay on the diet. This man had exhausted himself by fighting (and eventually losing) a battle with an enemy that didn't even exist.

Food Control Training is not deprivation. Living thin does not mean living without. The feelings of deprivation that you may have experienced on past diets were a product of a mind-set you imposed on *yourself.* No one was depriving you. You did not check your free will at the door when you signed up for the diet program. Your food options were—and are—always open.

The winners at weight loss know this instinctively because they've already eaten it all. They know that when they were eating it all they were not happy, they were miserable. The more they ate, the worse they felt and the worse they looked. That life (of being fat and out of control) was not some mythological paradise and the winners never forget that. They don't surrender their free will when they go on a diet, they take it with them. When they are faced with a trigger food, they don't say, "Oh, gee, I really want it, but I can't!" They say, "Sure, I *can* have it, but I choose not to.

It's not worth it—it's not worth being fat." They know, from experience, that only the thin say, "No, thank you."

Don't be tripped up by the fact that you may not always feel happy about saying this. No one is always happy about what they have to do to make their lives better. But they are happi*er* for having done it.

BEWARE THE "POOR ME" SYNDROME

When it comes to food, most of us still seem to feel that we are the center of the universe. We think we should be able to eat it all without having to pay any price. And when anyone reminds us that thin is not free—that we cannot eat it all and still be thin—we become indignant. We think, "Poor me, that's so unfair!"

The "Poor Me" Syndrome is the ultimate in the deprivation mind-set. It not only says you are deprived, it says you have a *right* to feel that way. It puts the blame for your weight problem squarely outside of yourself and onto the vagaries of an unjust world. In the process, it strips you of any control over your own body.

Feeling deprived is really just another way of surrendering to the control of food. It is a denial of your freedom and self-determination. You don't need a diet or a doctor to control your food intake. You have the knowledge and power to do that all on your own. You simply need to use it.

Good food is one of life's great pleasures. Sharing a meal with the people we love is one of the most enjoyable experiences any of us can have. But food should *enhance* life; it should not be the centerpiece of a life. Your life should not be controlled by food any more than it should be controlled by drugs or alcohol or any other external substance. You cannot focus your life on food and be thin. Being a foodie

---

is antagonistic to living thin. If getting control of your life and weight are your goals, then you have to pick what is important to you and go with it.

The beauty behind this deal is that once you make the decision, life becomes so much easier. Dieters spend so much time worrying about their failing willpower, they don't see that *control power* is more important than *willpower.* Once you master control, each day is no longer a continuing battle requiring willpower because the new way of eating and thinking about food becomes as automatic and natural as breathing.

The next time you are faced with a trigger food and find yourself feeling sorry for yourself, stop! Don't exhaust yourself by fighting imaginary enemies. Pull yourself together and make your choice. Decide whether you are going to walk away or exercise your option to eat that food—with full knowledge that if you eat it you'll have to wear it. Whatever your choice, take responsibility for it—don't blame the diet, or the food, or the argument you had twenty minutes before. Don't complain about your weight and bore everyone with talk of how you're going to go on a diet.

Thin is not a birthright. Neither is being able to have anything you want anytime you want. If you want to be thin, you must occasionally say no. And if you are going to say no you have to do it of your own free will. Such *self-chosen avoidance* isn't deprivation, it's liberation. And with each "No, thank you" you will gain a little more control, self-reliance, and self-esteem.

Myth 2: Doing Without Hurts

When I am interviewed about Food Control Training, reporters frequently ask, "But isn't it impossible?" Their incredulousness shows that they have fallen victim to the second deprivation myth—that it is impossible to do without something you once loved. But nothing could be further from the truth.

Time and avoidance change many things, including food preferences. Your Eating Print has revealed the food preferences that need to change but haven't. You know which of your favorite treats have outlived their usefulness in your life. These trigger foods have no place in your new life of thin. Remember, the reason you are passing up these foods is because they have caused a problem in your life. Eating them was not a paradise, it was responsible for misery. Not eating them can only make things better.

Besides, you've already tasted it all, there are no more surprises. You know the taste and texture of virtually every treat imaginable—what more can it give you? Think of it like a businessperson: It's simply not a good trade-off. It's not a good deal.

The evidence of the Eating Print is irrefutable. If you haven't been able to control a particular food in all the years you've tried to lose weight, do not torture yourself with talk of "I'll just have a little." With these foods, it is actually *easier* to pass up the food entirely than to try to have a little. Where there cannot be *moderation,* there must be *elimination.* (And there cannot be equivocation, for ambivalence is the core of lapsing back into the old patterns.)

I can think of nothing more masochistic than tasting a trigger food, reactivating all the old urges and cravings, and then trying to be satisfied with a little bit when you know there is more there just waiting to be eaten. *That* is what leads to feelings of deprivation. *That* is what leads to despair and to binge eating. Simply say that this food is not for me, it is not worth the chaos and the weight gain that it will bring into my life.

CALORIES ARE NOT CREATED EQUAL ✧ THINK OF YOUR CALORIES LIKE

Just as former smokers recognize that they cannot have just one cigarette and recovering alcoholics recognize that they cannot have just one glass of wine, you must recognize the foods you cannot control. Don't torture yourself by trying to eat limited portions of a food that triggers all your most compulsive eating behaviors. After all, there are thousands of delicious foods out there that won't put you at war with yourself. Learn to appreciate and enjoy them, and let your old trigger foods go.

Granted, forgoing an ice cream sundae may be hard at first. But the initial resistance won't last forever. The pull you have for it today will not be the same six months or even a month from now. If you ask a former smoker how she felt when she was smoking, she'll probably say she couldn't imagine life without cigarettes. Ask how she felt during the first weeks after quitting, and she'll probably admit she was climbing the walls. But if you ask how she feels *today,* you will hear how it is to walk without feeling winded, to have clothes that no longer smell like ashtrays, to have hundreds of extra dollars to spend each year. She won't tell you that she is deprived. On the contrary, she'll probably say she wishes she'd never started smoking. That's how it is with letting go of your trigger foods. It may be difficult at first, but the long-term benefits far outweigh any short-term discomforts. I (and my clients) have found that it is easier to say "no" than to just have a little.

Myth 3: Doing Without Is Abnormal

Frequently, I hear people say, "Oh, but I just want to be able to eat normally." I remind them that being fat isn't a normal condition. And I wish for them that they can live their lives at a normal weight. I wish that for you. That is far more important than worrying about what the next person is eating or what they think about what you're eating.

Myth 4: If You Can't Have It, You'll Binge

The same people who cannot imagine saying good-bye to their favorite foods usually believe that they will go off the deep end and binge if they try to totally avoid those foods. Even some health professionals fall for this myth. After all, they say, forbidden fruit is always the most seductive. But what they don't seem to get is that for tens of millions of us, having a little is much harder than having none. That's why we freely choose to strive for this goal. It is not imposed on us by some higher power or authority, causing us to rebel like an adolescent with food.

They have got it backward. For most of us, bingeing has nothing to do with avoidance. It has everything to do with availability! Trigger foods that are available, that you allow yourself to have, are the ones you will find yourself bingeing on. That's why you have a problem with weight in the first place. You binged on the same foods time and time again.

The ultimate deflation of this myth came about in the past few years when food producers started to make fat-free cookies, cakes, crackers, and other snack foods that were previously forbidden because of their calories and fat content. Now, at last, paradise had arrived, these foods weren't forbidden! In fact, many were advertised as "guilt-free." They were considered safe. They were considered healthy. People who had problems with the high-fat variety felt they had found a cure, they could now go out and buy the low-fat/no-fat varieties and have it both ways—eat their favorite foods and still be thin.

But they were wrong. These misguided men and women soon discovered that they were abusing their no-fat saviors—just as much as they were the high-fat ones. The bingeing was inherent in the food and its interaction with their biology, it had nothing to do with whether they had tried to avoid the foods or not. This is why almost all of my clients now agree with this guiding principle: If you abuse the high-calorie/high-fat variety, you'll abuse the low-cal/low-fat variety, perhaps even more.

For some, "forbidden" may be the same as "seductive," it's true. There is a subgroup of food-oriented people with whom, because of their previous conditioning, dieting can prompt an Adam and Eve Complex. Like the residents of the Garden of Eden, these food-centered individuals pine after their lost treats until it all becomes too much and they plunge back into their old habits—and their old weight.

What these people will be happy to learn is that in Food Control Training there is no such thing as a forbidden fruit. No one is threatening you with expulsion from paradise. You and you alone decide what foods you can and cannot control. You choose the foods that you will abstain from, limit, or continue to eat without limitations based on the lessons of your Eating Print, not the arbitrary word of some diet expert.

Myth 5: You'll Never Enjoy Food Again!

This is the deprivation myth that I am particularly tired of hearing. For the record: Healthy foods do not have to be bland, low-calorie foods are not tasteless, and living by your Eating Print does not mean abandoning everything you ever loved in the world of food. There are whole schools of cooking—from the nouvelle cuisine of France to the new "light" cuisine of California—that are based on healthy, low-fat foods. You can eat out and eat well at gourmet restaurants the world over and still maintain food control.

The great irony of our foodie culture is that it has such an extraordinarily limited imagination. Most modern Americans rely on a very small, very dull, and not particularly healthy assortment of foods that they eat over and over again—the same few vegetables, the same few meats, and the same snack foods that satisfy an eat-and-run lifestyle. Despite the fact that we can buy practically any food—no matter how exotic or out of season—at any time of the day or night, few of us venture beyond the limits of our favorite foods.

"But I can't live without them! I can't live without them!" That is what the deprivationists would have you believe. They claim the lure of these morsels is so powerful that trying to eat without them is like trying to breathe without air. But the foods that this society considers so vital— the sweets and snack foods that so many people live for— did not even exist for most of human history. There are entire societies that live perfectly well without the "benefits" of chips, dips, double cheeseburgers, french fries, cookies, or M&Ms. Indeed, for almost all of human history, the overwhelming majority of humankind has never seen, tasted, or wanted these foods. There is nothing inherent in these tastes that is critical to human survival.

Even in countries where such treats are popular, there have always been men and women who have abstained. Some abstain for medical reasons, knowing that eating certain foods can mean illness or even death. Others abstain for religious reasons, following the tenets of their faith out of a devotion to a higher good. Whatever the reason, however, all of these people live full, productive lives.

When you decide it's time to let go of some of those troublesome old favorites of yours, you will discover something wonderful: There is a virtually unlimited selection of foods out there that are healthy, low-fat, *and* delicious to eat. You don't need to be a Cordon Bleu chef to enjoy them. You don't need a state-of-the-art kitchen. All you need is a willingness to go beyond the limits of your old eating habits. In Part Three, you'll find the information you need. And once you've expanded your cooking horizons, you'll discover it's almost impossible to feel satisfied within the limited boundaries of your old trigger foods.

Ideally, the combination of these new foods and a new perspective on the "bad old" foods should be enough to quell any longings for your triggers. But I understand that we don't live in an ideal world. I also understand that giving up *all* of your triggers *all* of the time can, for some people, seem nearly impossible. Some people can get so discouraged, they'll give up on all the other strategies they've mastered. I tell those individuals that not every trigger is a problem in every situation. For some triggers, there is a healthy, controlled alternative to total avoidance. If you have one or two trigger foods that you would like to keep in your life, you can do it—if you're careful.

Boxing It In

One of my clients is a middle-aged attorney named Gilbert. When I first met Gil he had a list of trigger foods and situations as long as his arm. Over the course of two years he managed to get all of them under control—except one.

Gil's problem trigger is a rich, flaky confection called rugelah. He loves it. Left to his own devices, he would happily eat his way through an entire bakery. He's tried to go

WHEN IS DEPRIVATION NOT DEPRIVATION?

Have you ever bought something you had to scrimp and save for? Perhaps you bought it on layaway or saved up for months. How did you feel when you bought it and finally brought it home? Did you look at your now empty bank account and say, "Oh no, I'm financially deprived"?

If anything, you probably looked from that empty bank account to your new car, house, or vacation tickets and felt positively privileged. It was a sign of achievement, of success, of a job well done. You may have spent months or even years saying "No, thank you" to dozens of minor pleasures, but it was all worth it because you knew the prize you were aiming for.

Deprivation is all a matter of perspective. When you say "no" to one of your triggers, you aren't saying "no" to happiness. You are saying "yes" to a healthy, thinner you. You are saying "yes" to a longer, more vital life. You are saying "yes" to all of the clothes, events, and activities that you have had to avoid for years because of your weight.

So when it comes time to take your eyes off the dessert cart, keep your eyes on the prize—the image of yourself as you've always wanted to be—slender, smiling, fit.

cold turkey, and he's decided that he simply does not want to do it.

This doesn't mean Gil has resigned himself to spending the rest of his life fat. On the contrary, he's absolutely committed to maintaining his healthy weight. But he has arrived at a compromise with his most persistent trigger—one that allows him to enjoy it on occasion without losing control. He has mastered the art of boxing it in.

Rugelah is a classic holiday food. Gil's compromise is a simple one. He allows himself to enjoy rugelah—as much as he wants—at two parties each holiday season, no more, no less. He doesn't buy it the rest of the year; he never has it at home, but he enjoys it to the fullest at his two allowed parties. He has moments of wanting it at other times, but they're bearable because he knows he'll have his chance later.

Another client found a clever way to use his maintenance calories—the additional calories he could include once he had reached his goal weight. Although he had a history of eating more than one roll when the bread basket came around, it was also the food he missed the most while losing weight. So we struck a caloric bargain: He would continue to eat the low-calorie, low-fat restaurant entrées he had been eating during weight loss and use his maintenance calories for one or two rolls whenever he went to his favorite restaurant. I must note, however, that this is not a route I advocate for all of my clients. This is an exceptionally honest and determined human being, and what works for him may not work for any number of others.

I do a little boxing in myself. Generally, I try to steer clear of fancy desserts. But when I visit my sisters, who are great cooks, for the holidays, I allow myself to partake of the traditional dishes and the Italian pastries and other desserts that are always on hand—it's once a year and I know I can handle that. Many of my clients also practice boxing in on Thanksgiving or for the annual family picnic. Or those who find that they abuse the bread basket steer clear of it in restaurants but enjoy a bagel on Saturday mornings. Some of my New York clients who are very fond of steak will never eat it in a regular restaurant but will restrict it to special occasions when they go to New York City's famed steak house Peter Luger's. Others will eat cake only at specific birthday celebrations. Whatever the food, they don't deny that it is a pleasurable experience, but they don't fall into the trap of calling it a reward for living their life in a healthy manner. After all, it's not what you eat on a holiday or special occasion that makes you fat (as long as what you eat on the holiday or vacation *doesn't carry over* and influence what you will eat the next day and each day thereafter), but what you eat and bring into your home each day.

Maybe your "can't-live-without-it" trigger is ice cream. Maybe it's french fries. Whatever it is, take a look at your overall Eating Print and figure out where and when it is least likely to be a problem. Do you lose control when this food is in the house? Then *never* eat it when you're at home. Are you able to have "just a little" if you eat it at a restaurant? Then limit your consumption to occasions when you are dining out. And limit those occasions to special events or places, to prevent the F/Q Principle from going into effect. Limiting frequency is essential, since, according to that principle, the *F* comes first.

By boxing in your trigger to specific, carefully limited situations, you can have the best of both worlds—an occasional taste of one of your old favorites without the loss of control. Boxing it in works only with trigger foods that are indeed controllable. If you have a trigger food that always sends you into a tailspin, it's not a candidate for boxing in. As always, when choosing your "boxable" foods, absolute honesty is required. Otherwise, they will box you in to a life of fat.

When You Can't Have Everything You Want, You Can Still Have Everything You Need!

Most dieters approach weight loss with a prison mentality. They look upon the diet as time served and, when done, they can't wait to go back to their old ways, to indulging in the foods they were "deprived" of during the diet.

If you go into your weight-loss program with such an attitude, the real prison time will come *after* the diet is over—when you step back into the prison of your triggers and once again fall under the control of food. Foods cannot possess you, seduce you, or deprive you of your free will. The only power they have is the power you give them. And whenever you turn that power over to food, you are depriving yourself of the right to be thin, the right to be healthy and fit, the right to own the clothes you want and to look the way you want to look. *That* is the real deprivation.

Letting go of the deprivation mind-set is a major step forward on the road to your permanent thin. But it's only a beginning. Even under the best of circumstances, the old beliefs and feelings of deprivation will sometimes resurface, pounding at your resolve. To combat those waves of deprivation, you will need to let go of the whole language of "goodies" and "treats" and replace it with new, more functional talk.

It is never enough to "just say no." You need to have something to say "yes" to. If you want to stop going to food when you are upset, you need to have somewhere else to go. Similarly, if you are going to give up your old food talk and, with it, deprivation, you had better write yourself a new script. And the best script is saying "yes" to a thin and healthy you.

STEP FOUR
CHANGING YOUR
"FOOD TALK"

*It takes two to speak the truth—one
to speak, and another to hear.*
HENRY DAVID THOREAU

We all talk to ourselves. We may not want to admit it but all thinking human beings have a constant stream-of-consciousness chatter going on. In fact, if you've ever been on a diet, you've probably had entire conversations just about dessert, conversations that probably went something like this: "Gosh, that looks delicious! . . . (But what about my diet?) . . . I'll have them hold the whipped cream . . . (Sure, that will save some calories!) . . . and I won't finish these potatoes . . . (I'll probably be too full to eat dinner later anyway!) . . . It's been *such* a miserable day . . . (Everyone deserves a treat now and then) . . ." *"Oh, waiter!* Will you bring the dessert cart around?"

Sometimes these conversations may end on a different note. Instead of calling for dessert you motion for the check. Instead of leaving the restaurant feeling guilty and satiated you leave feeling righteous and frustrated. But whatever the outcome, the basic script is the same—full of longing for, and idealization of, food.

These internal dialogues—the snatches of thought that seem to come from nowhere—are your Food Talk. Food Talk is like a cassette tape inside your brain filled with the messages and food beliefs that were passed on to you by your parents, your culture, and your long-dead ancestors. Whenever you are near food, particularly your trigger foods, the tape switches on. And if you've got a weight problem, you can be certain that a lot of the messages it contains are destructive. They are encouraging your foodie mind-set, fostering your feelings of deprivation, and eroding your control over food. It's time to get in there and change that tape!

Most of my clients find it easy to see the absurdity of the deprivation mind-set when they are talking with me in my office. They recognize that their trigger foods are enemies, not treats. They know that the real deprivation is in never living thin. They see that their old foodie beliefs were irrational, illogical, and destructive. On a conscious level, they make the shift from foodie to realist in only a few sessions. But that conscious shift needs reinforcement.

Food Talk isn't conscious. It is not rational. It was "taped" long before your logical thinking processes were even developed, and it has been reinforced ever since. It strikes without warning and often without your being aware of it. As a result, even the most conscientious dieters find themselves thinking, "Wouldn't that be delicious!" when they know perfectly well it will *not* be delicious in the long run—it will only be fattening.

The Food Talk of those who succeed at weight loss, however, is very different from the Food Talk of those who valiantly try but fail. In years of studying the thought patterns of people who succeed at weight loss, I have discovered that the Food Talk of the winners is almost entirely free of foodie messages. They have made a *cognitive switch* in their self-talk about food. Their internal dialogue is full of supportive, positive messages about their bodies, their health, and their sense of control over their lives. They don't fall for the Great Lie ("I'll just have a little!"). They don't negotiate with food. And most importantly, they don't berate or abuse themselves. Simply put, the Food Talk of the winners is *motivating,* not demoralizing. Faced with the Great Lie, they dare to talk back.

Your Food Talk can help you or hinder you. Indeed, it can be the difference between success and failure. It can speed you along the road away from the deprivation mindset and foodie-ism, or it can drag you back and keep you enslaved to your trigger foods. The choice is yours. Because with time—and practice—you can rerecord your internal tape and free yourself from the old Food Talk. But first, you'll have to identify the messages that are undermining your control.

Identifying Your Food Talk

Rewriting your Food Talk—the fourth step that leads to successful weight loss—means changing your head as well as your weight. Food Talk is rarely as obvious as the fictional conversation at the beginning of this chapter. Many Food Talk messages are *subliminal*—you feel them and respond to them, but you aren't consciously aware of hearing them. To counter these subtle messages, you need to drag them out into the light of day, and the easiest way to do that is with a little free association.

Go back to the list of trigger foods that you made on page 43. On a separate sheet of paper, for each individual food, write down the first ten words or phrases that come to your mind about that food. If possible, have a friend read your trigger list to you so that you are responding to a verbal cue.

Write down whatever comes into your mind, as it comes into your mind. *Don't edit yourself.* If the first word that comes into your mind when you think of champagne is *sex,* go ahead and write it down. If you can't think of ten words or phrases, fine. There are no right or wrong answers. You are simply trying to get a handle on what you really think and feel about these foods.

Once you've gone through all of your trigger foods, take a look at the words you used. Is there a pattern? Are your food phrases

- about the food's taste and texture (rich, creamy, luscious, and so on)?
- about how the food makes you feel (comforted, exhilarated, satisfied, sexy)?
- food-glorifying (heavenly, perfect, scrumptious, the best, and so on)?

The words you chose are at the heart of your Food Talk. They are the messages you receive whenever you are in the presence of these foods. And more than likely, they have very little to do with the reality of these foods in your life.

For example, consider the words that one of my clients wrote in response to the word *chocolate—mousse, pudding, heaven, happiness, rich, comfort, freedom, milk, delicious, perfect.* This woman had been at least 50 pounds overweight for more than fifteen years. She had spent thousands of dollars on diet plans and thrown away entire wardrobes when she gained the weight back. She was the first to admit that her problem was chocolate. She knew that whenever she returned to eating chocolate she lost control over food and gained weight. But even with this knowledge, when she heard the word *chocolate* most of her responses were positively adoring.

This client, like all the winners at weight loss, eventually erased most of those responses from her internal tape and replaced them with realistic, positive messages that enabled her to say no to chocolate without feeling depressed and deprived. How? Through a technique called Cognitive Switching.

Cognitive Switching

Cognitive Switching is a simple process of *replacement* and *repetition*—replacement of the old Food Talk phrases with new, functional messages and a repetition of these new phrases so that they become part of your unconscious.

To do Cognitive Switching, you need a few simple, inexpensive tools: a tape recorder, some cassettes, a portable tape player (like a Walkman), and, of course, your knowledge of your Food Talk and its roots.

You weren't born with negative Food Talk. It takes outside influences—advertising, school lunches, trick-or-treating, birthday parties—to make children sugar fiends and junk food junkies. And your inner language reflects that.

The Food Talk that feels as much a part of you as your blood type is really a mix of *other* voices—the well-meaning voices of your parents or grandparents, the voices of Madison Avenue advertising executives, the voices of ancient ancestors who lived in fear of deprivation, and the voice of a primitive, petulant, and remarkably persistent part of your psyche that Sigmund Freud would have called the id.

The id is the most primal aspect of your being, interested only in immediate gratification and quick satisfaction. It is impulse central. The id is the ultimate spoiled child. It isn't interested in your high blood pressure. It doesn't care about the bulge in your waistline or the bloat in your face. It doesn't care about your cholesterol level. It's not concerned with the fact that you find it difficult to climb the stairs. It just knows what it wants and it wants it *now!*

In most aspects of your life, you keep the id in check fairly well. You may *want* to throw your neighbor's stereo out of the nearest window, but you don't actually go over and do it. You have a system of personal and social checks and balances that reminds you to rein in those impulses.

No such system exists for food. The lessons you were taught by your parents, society at large, and even your genetic code all say that *food is good.* So your id, reinforced by all that programming, runs rampant every time you are faced with your triggers. It starts playing that old Food Talk tape at top volume—demanding the foods you most want to avoid and blocking your memories of how much trouble those foods caused you in the past.

In the moments when your negative Food Talk seems to be screaming most loudly, it helps to remember just where that Food Talk originates. Before you surrender to those impulses, before you accept their false promises and specious logic, ask yourself, Do you really want to take orders from these people?

- Do you really want to be ruled by the fears of ancestors who died thousands of years ago?
- Do you really want to be jerked around by the capricious impulses of your id?
- Do you really want to fall for the promises of purveyors of junk food, who neither know nor care about your weight problem?

Of course not. That's why you're going to make the cognitive switch.

Making the Cognitive Switch

Foods have no power of their own. They can't hypnotize you. They can't mesmerize you. They can't pull a gun on you and force you to devour them.

Any hypnotic power that foods hold over you is the power that you have given them. You mesmerize yourself by saying the wrong things to yourself about food and by listening to the messages of your id and the foodie value system. Every time you tell yourself, "Oh, I have to have it!" you are reinforcing the backward value system that got you into trouble in the first place. It's a process of self-hypnosis: We come to need what we tell ourselves we need. It's an internal advertising campaign for the food.

Cognitive Switching gives you an ad campaign for health and long-term happiness. By giving you powerful campaign slogans or aphorisms—something like *"I don't take the first little taste . . . I don't begin. I don't have any problem"*—it turns you around so you're facing forward, not backward, so you can get on with the business of enjoying a life free from the domination of food.

Over many years of working with the winners to rerecord their internal tapes, I have come up with a list of healthy slogans that you can use to replace ones that have been causing you to fail. Many of them come directly from my clients, for after talking to literally thousands of men and women in the course of my work, I realized that the winners seemed to share a common language. Those who lost the weight and kept it off spoke to themselves with key messages. These are the new messages that you can record on your internal tape.

You do not have to stick to these words and phrases verbatim if you don't want to. In fact, when you record your actual tapes—and I will tell you how to do just that right here, right now—you can and should use your own words, concoct your own aphorisms geared to your own needs. Use the cognitive switches listed in the box that begins below as a guide, and be as creative as you want.

Cognitive Switching is like an "off" switch. When a harmful thought from the foodie culture slips into your brain, your mind will spit the old thought out and replace it with a new phrase. Over time, this switching will become effortless. You won't have to consciously think, "Oh, now what was it that Dr. Gullo suggested I say?" It will just be there in your mind.

COGNITIVE SWITCH-OFFS

LOSERS	WINNERS
"Just one won't hurt."	"If I could just have one, I wouldn't have been fat for the last ten years!"
	"One was never enough before. It won't be enough now."

LOSERS	WINNERS
"I'll just have one peanut."	"Stop lying—in twenty years, I haven't been able to have one."
	"I've gained more weight with my fingers than with my mouth!"
"Oh, I can eat extra, the label says *no fat*."	"No fat doesn't mean *not fattening*."
	"It doesn't say *no calories*."
"I paid for it, I might as well eat it."	"Calories cost more than dollars—you have to wear them."
	"If I eat it, I have to wear it."
"It's only 20 calories."	"It's not how many calories but how many I'll eat."
	"It's not the calories, but the calorie units that count."
"It's a sin to waste food."	"It's a greater sin to waste my body and my life."
	"It's a greater sin to make myself fat."
	"It's a sin to raise my blood pressure."
	"It's a sin to clog my arteries."
	"It's a sin to die before my time because of a few calories."
"I hate to throw food out."	"Better to put it in the garbage pail than become the garbage pail."

LOSERS	WINNERS
	"Protecting my body is more important than protecting my leftovers."
"Oh, it smells so good."	"So good? That's the smell of fat."
"Oh, this food tastes so good, I can never get enough of it."	"Why not be honest—stop calling it a food. Call it what it really is—an appetite-stimulant pill."
"I blew it with the french fries, I might as well have the ice cream."	"There's no such thing as blowing it."
	"What's done is done. Let go of it and move on."
	"Don't use one mistake as an excuse to make others."
	"The sooner I stop, the less I'll have to wear tomorrow."
"I deserve a treat."	"I deserve to be thin."
	"Losing weight is a better treat."
	"Don't settle so cheaply. I deserve a healthy life of thin."
"It's been such a stressful day."	"It's more stressful to be fat!"
"I'm feeling so blue."	"Food won't help. Happy or sad, it's better being thin!"
	"Eating doesn't erase feeling, it just makes you feel worse."

LOSERS	WINNERS
"I've been so good, I deserve a reward."	"Living thin is the best reward." "I don't reward myself with things that cause me pain."
"I feel so frustrated, I could devour everything in sight!"	"If I devour it, fat will devour me!"
"It looks so good!"	"It's not how it looks on the plate or the table, but how it looks on me." "Not on my thighs it doesn't!" "It looks like every other food that made me fat." "What's so 'good' about it? It's given me obesity, hypertension, and misery." "I don't like it enough to wear it!"
"I just can't resist."	"I've come too far to take orders from a cookie!" "I do not negotiate with baked goods!"
"It's so hard to say no."	"Only the thin say 'No, thank you.'"
"I love pizza."	"It's better to wear Italian than to eat it!"
"When I see it, I crave it."	"I don't take the first little taste . . . I don't begin, I don't have any problem."

ARE HEAVY FROM WHAT THEY EAT BEFORE, AFTER, AND IN BETWEEN

LOSERS	WINNERS
	"Cravings are feelings, not commands."
	"It's just a feeling. I'm not bleeding, there is no pain, I don't need to call 911 for the rescue squad."
	"Cravings last only a few minutes. Thin is worth a few minutes!"
	"Stop looking at it—what are you looking at? You already see it every day on your thighs."
"It's not fair that I can't have dessert!"	"I *can* have dessert. I *choose* not to!"
	"It's not fair that I've spent the last ten years being fat because of dessert!"
	"It would be more unfair never to be thin."
	"When I *was* eating desserts I was fat and miserable."
"I can't deprive my family of their treats."	"I won't deprive my family of their health."
"But it's on sale!"	"No sale is more important than my body, my health, and my right to be thin."
	"Thin begins in the supermarket."
	"If I don't buy it, I don't have to wear it."

LOSERS	WINNERS
"It's free, I might as well eat it."	"Calories aren't free—you have to wear them."
"I'm on vacation—I should be able to eat what I want."	"I've taken a vacation from good judgment with my eating for years, I don't need another seven days."
"I've been doing everything right and still haven't lost the weight—what's the use?"	"It took years to gain this weight—why can't I be patient with my body a few more days?"

These Food Talk exercises are a friendly tap on the shoulder when you most need it, gentle reminders of what the food *really* means in your life. They are like a friend nudging you and saying, "Uh, excuse me, but don't you remember what happened the last time you ate that food?"

Recording Your Own Internal Tape

No health professional or therapist—no matter how devoted—can be with a client twenty-four hours a day. That's why I want you to make some portable reinforcers—cassette tapes of the key phrases that you most need to hear and internalize. These cassettes are your pocket cheering section, ready-made advocates that are always there to give you support whenever you might need it. They can be popped in a Walkman for a run around the park or played over your car's speakers on the way to work. They provide a comprehensive support system that you can draw on at any time to help eradicate the old Food Talk and reinforce the new.

Your Food Talk tapes should be as individual as you are. They should speak to your personal strengths, your unique accomplishments, and your most treasured goals. They should make you feel good about the work you are doing and encourage you to do more. Basically, your Food Talk tapes are an advertising campaign. The product they are pitching is the new, thin, healthy you. And like any successful ad campaign, they need to be upbeat, catchy, and full of powerful images that will capture your imagination and interest.

You may feel a bit awkward at first as you speak into the tape recorder. But like so many aspects of Food Control Training, the consistent and faithful repetition of the process makes it easier and easier to do.

As you listen to the tapes with increasing regularity, your mind will start reinforcing the messages on its own and your thought patterns will begin to mimic the ideas on the tapes. After just a few weeks of daily listening, you should begin to hear the words of your new Food Talk even when you aren't listening to the tapes. The process of repetition will begin to change that internal tape, and the changes will be seen not only in your attitude, but in your behavior with food.

I am providing the scripts of a few sample tapes that you can use to get started. These scripts can be tailored to suit your own situation. Feel free to alter anything that you don't feel comfortable saying. You may find it more powerful to speak in the first person, saying, "I will start my Food Control Plan today." Or if cheerleading works better for you, you might consider the second-person tense: "*You* will start your Food Control Plan today." And later you may want to write your own scripts entirely.

TAPE 1: GETTING STARTED

I will start my Food Control Plan today. I will not put it on hold. I don't have to wait till the start of a new month, I don't have to wait till after the big luncheon next week, I don't have to wait. I won't say, "I'll start eating well tomorrow!" How long have I had this weight problem? Ten years? Twenty years? And I'm still saying tomorrow?

Saying tomorrow is saying a lie. If I can come up with an excuse for not starting today, what makes me think I won't have another excuse tomorrow, the following tomorrow, and the tomorrow after that? Saying tomorrow is saying I will *not* do it today.

Today I will start living as I never have before. I will shop as never before. Remember, *if you don't buy it, you don't eat it.* As I carry the bags home, I will feel stronger than I ever have, I will feel the blood pumping through me, I will take deep invigorating breaths of air, stride through the parking lot, up the driveway, along the sidewalk, all the way home.

I will cook well because I have the skills, and I will feel good. There is nothing in the house that can trigger me. If there is anything in the house that can trigger me right now, then right after this recording ends I am going to take it and throw it away. That's right, as soon as this recording ends, I turn off the recorder and go straight into the kitchen, put the fattening things in the trash, tie up the plastic bag, and put it out for collection. If it's not in my kitchen, then it's not on my hips.

If I find myself thinking, obsessing, *missing* the food, I have a simple three-word magic pill: *Get over it.*

I can say that to myself any day, anytime, and laugh. And I can also say, don't whine about it, because then I make myself miserable, even though I don't eat anything. There's a whole world out there with AIDS, homelessness, and cancer. And I'm worrying about a piece of food?

Get over it. Move on. It's just a glob of calories.

Thinking is the first step toward the behavior. *Cut off* the thinking. *Don't allow* the thinking. I don't take the first little taste . . . I don't begin. I don't

---

have any problem. It's only a piece of food. And no matter what it is, *thin tastes better!*

What will make me be able to start and follow through with Food Control Training when previously I have failed on so many other programs? I didn't fail on those programs . . . those programs failed me because they weren't tailor-made for me like Food Control Training. And why will I keep going? Because, for once, I've got my headset on straight. I'm not doing it because someone else has told me to, I'm doing this because my own love and caring for myself won't allow me to live an unhealthy, unhappy life anymore.

Finally, I won't allow it, me, myself, I won't allow it any longer.

Life is short. The highest purpose of life is to function happily, to be happy. I can do that.

I won't say tomorrow.

Because I can do it . . . today.

TAPE 2: TURNING OFF THE DEPRIVATION SWITCH

It is so easy to lose my focus between what is essential and what is nonessential. Yet it looks like I am finding my way. I have restored the balance in my life. I have flipped off the switch that controls the feelings of deprivation in my head—and with that one flick of a switch, I can find my way to a new sense of happiness and control. I can achieve thin. Each time I say, "No, thank you," I say *yes* to thin.

That is the victory. *That* is why I feel good today and why I'm not worried if the scale goes down 3 pounds or 1^1/$_4$ pounds. For I know when I'm done that I have done the one thing I have never succeeded at doing, through all the diet plans and good intentions of the past. *That* is why I'm starting to feel confident . . . and I should feel confident.

Now think of the weeks ahead. If I find myself obsessing on a piece of food, I will say, "Get over it." Get over myself. Get over being a foodie. Remember that of all the things I want to do, all the places I want to go in life, there's one place I don't have to worry about: I don't ever have to visit Disneyland. I've been *living* in a Disneyland, thinking I could have it all and still be thin. And thinking that, in spite of all the blessings of life, if there is one thing from the world of food I cannot have, then that means I must be deprived. Taking orders from food is the real deprivation.

But I'm getting over that whole philosophy of life. I'm starting to live in the real world, where the most important thing is not *what I eat* for lunch or dinner today but how I live my life, today and every day.

In the perfect world, yes, I should be able to cook anything I want, taste anything. But the world is not perfect. I am not perfect, neither is Dr. Gullo, and we never will be. So I should start living with *who I am* rather than who I should be.

That's easy to forget when I'm at the party and the hors d'oeuvres are being passed around, or when the kids come home from school and I have to fix them a snack, or when I'm out on that big-deal business lunch and I am sitting within inches of the lethal bread basket. My greatest strength at any and all of these times, however—and I *know* it—is not beginning. Don't begin with the trigger foods, don't begin trigger behaviors, steer clear of trigger situations, and march away from trigger emotions. For once and for all, listen to your Eating Print, turn up the volume of your Eating Print, and drown out all the pleading and whining of the deprivationists of this world.

From the day that I let go of deprivation's greatest lie—that I can have just a little—from that day on, I'll start to live with honesty and integrity. I am who I am and the greatest diet in the world for me is to know myself—to know what I can handle and what I cannot handle, to understand when I lose the weight, I don't lose the problem. I have the same taste buds, I have the same personality.

But the good thing is, since I'm highly predictable, I know exactly what to expect. And it's highly controllable. That is why I'll be able to stop buying certain foods and making certain foods. When it comes to food, I can become as predictable and reliable as the laws of gravity.

Finally, I am opening my eyes and *seeing* it. I have all the answers already, I can say to myself. I can see that now. Because if I look back over the past years, it is the same foods, the same patterns, the same excuses, the same times of the day and week. Finally, I am able to see.

And I will see a new body. And I will be able to keep it this time.

I've finally come home. This is not a new me. This is *me* as I am right now, but minus the excuses and the foods that have been tripping me up. The new me is the old me . . . the only me . . . only better.

TAPE 3: MAINTENANCE AND THE REAL CLEARING

My success is measured best not by the scale but by individual clearings and breakthroughs. For I will not persevere or endure if I do not believe in *why* I am doing it. When I changed my dinner plans and my approach to cooking, preparing, and shopping for food, that was another breakthrough and clearing. It is more important how I treat my body and myself and my quality of life than how I treat my dinner parties. I'm reasserting the priorities of the values of life over cooking and food. It's not about deprivation, it's about being a selective gourmet.

My food, my dinner parties, what I wanted to cook, what I thought should be on the table, what I *had* to order at the restaurant came before any consideration of control, before any thought as to how much weight I would gain. I would completely turn off my good judgment. How could I possibly succeed going from weight program to weight program if I was a foodie and food was a principal value of my life?

Food is designed to enhance life and enrich it, not diminish it. The way I allowed food to rule my life was diminishing my life. But I have put my values in the right place once and for all. The deprivationist in me is losing its power and a new, thin, empowered self is emerging.

Most of all, I see something else emerging: I'm becoming a very good self-therapist. I talk to myself, nurture myself with my talking and caring, *not* with food. I'm reminding myself that *I* am much greater than this piece of food that sits on the plate before me. It's just a glob of calories. I don't take orders from a piece of food. Don't invest it with some kind of magical power and aura for happiness and problem solving. Food temptations are just feelings, not commands . . . they pass.

Now I can see the whole mosaic. I have nothing against any specific foods if I can live with them in harmony. But if I cannot, then they are wrong for my shopping cart, for my home, for my life. Because life and the quality of living come first. I am simply reasserting the correct values of what works for me.

Now think of the weeks ahead. We have finally agreed when there is a collision between a food and my critical life goals, we don't throw out the goals, we throw out the food. They are not in the same league . . . they are not even *close*.

Besides, I'll never have to worry about saying, "Uh, I missed out on this or that," because I've already eaten it. I've already eaten enough in my lifetime for five lifetimes of food. I've had enough food curiosity to last a century. I've read enough, thought enough, and fantasized enough. My life has had too much food in it, not too little, and I'm running around fearing I might be deprived of food?

That's the old thinking. That's yesterday's news. I was in complete denial. Now I know that I was being deprived of *life* because I was so worried about *food*. The very foodies who have never had a little keep deluding themselves that they will just have a little. . . . They are still around me now, they can still exert a power over me, subtly, imperceptibly, till I suddenly find myself thinking that maybe "just a little" is reasonable or possible.

Remember that. Remember that maintaining my weight doesn't mean giving up all I learned when I was losing weight. Maintaining weight means refreshing my memory every so often, keeping all I've learned in the forefront of my mind, pulling it out and mentally exercising with it just as I am

> physically exercising my limbs and muscles to keep them as toned and trim and healthy-looking as possible.
>
> I'll never entertain in the same way again. I'll never shop or cook in the same way . . . I will always live more protectively and with more care.
>
> That is the great victory.

Some Pointers and Practical How-tos

If you decide to try your hand at writing your own scripts, observe these basic guidelines.

Stick to the Point. Before you begin recording, write some scripts (or at least outlines of the points you want to cover). Keep them succinct and clear. Let each tape address a specific situation, belief, or trigger that is your particular problem. Label the tape accordingly.

Keep It Positive. Statements like "I deserve something better than a handful of calories and a few grams of fat" are considerably better than "Get that out of your mouth, you fat slob!" And if you find yourself at a loss for (positive) words, you can always rely on the ultimate truth, that no matter what the food or situation, "Thin tastes better!"

Keep It Short. Ideally, each tape should have only three to ten minutes' worth of talk on each side. Remember, the frequency of listening is the important part. If a tape is so long that it bores you, it won't do you any good. Five or six minutes is the average for most of my clients.

Reinforce Your Goals. Describe yourself in the clothes you've always wanted. Describe the "you, only better" that you envisioned when setting your weight goal.

Add Punch and Power. Remind yourself of the downside of your so-called goodies. Repeat the lessons of your Eating Print: List your trigger foods, behaviors, situations, and emotions. Remind yourself of the highest weight that you reached when you went back to these patterns. Repeat all the Great Lies you've told yourself and make the cognitive switches that sound right to you.

Look to the Future. When reminding yourself of the embarrassment and pain you endured from your old behavior, always bring it back to the benefits you'll enjoy from the new.

Emphasize Strength and Mastery. Speak in firm, assertive, and resolute tones. Remind yourself of your power and accomplishments in other aspects of your life. Don't beat yourself up. Guilt doesn't burn calories. Appeal to the motivating force that drives you—you feel miserable, your energy is too low, you're concerned about your health—whatever it may be.

Rehearse! Use the tapes to prepare for upcoming events. Is there an important business lunch coming up? Is it the week of the garden club bazaar, where everyone brings homemade cookies and strudels and cake? Describe the situation and how you will handle it. Paint a vivid picture and take yourself through every possible eventuality. Rehearse how you will say, "No, thank you," if offered a trigger food.

Give Them a "Soundtrack." Try recording one in your backyard, with the sounds of birds chirping and breezes blowing. Or play one of your favorite instrumental pieces. Be creative and have fun with it. The more entertaining they are, the more you'll want to listen.

Use a "Guest Artist." If you dislike the sound of your own voice (as many people do) ask a friend to do a guest appearance on your tapes. Ask someone whose voice you trust and enjoy. If you know someone who sounds like James Earl Jones, get him!

Use the Associative Edge. Some voices have more emotional resonance and significance than others. Advertising executives know this—that's why so many commercials feature grandfatherly old men or cute little kids. You can make use of the same technique in your tapes. For example, one of my clients had his seven-year-old son read some of his new aphorisms. It gave the boy a chance to practice his reading, and the father a chance to hear the most influential person in his life—his son—speaking to him about his health and well-being.

End on a High Note. When you feel yourself running out of steam, you can always have a rousing finish by concluding with the power statement "I don't take the first little taste, I don't begin. I don't have any problem."

Please Don't Squeeze the . . . Cellulite?

I have always been amazed at the powers of advertising. It can get us to buy just about *anything*. That's why I have tried to adapt the principles of advertising psychology to weight control. It had never been done before but, then again, for most people, attaining a lasting thin had never been done before either.

I believe those powers can work for you . . . if you make a tape. Don't say you feel silly. Just think . . .

- Please don't squeeze the Charmin.
- Plop, plop, fizz, fizz, oh what a relief it is.
- Fly the friendly skies.
- M&Ms melt in your mouth, not in your hand.

Most people remember the catchy, sometimes silly advertising slogans of their youth. And why not? That's the whole point: finding a word, phrase, or musical tag that is so distinctive, it's forever linked to a particular product.

Your new Food Talk and the tapes that reinforce it serve the same purpose. You want to come up with the words, phrases, and images that will evoke visions of the new, thin, healthy you. Many of my clients turn foodie advertising slogans on their ears, saying "Snickers *disappoints* you" instead of "Snickers satisfies you" or "M&Ms melt on your *thighs*" instead of "M&Ms melt in your mouth."

Some Final Advice

Once you've got your library of Food Talk tapes, make sure you listen to them every day. Listen to one on your Walkman while you're shopping, making dinner, or cleaning the house. And *always* listen to one before the situations (dinner parties, a weekend business trip, your favorite restaurant) when you have the most problems. To borrow a phrase from one of the world's most successful advertising campaigns, "Don't leave home without them!"

Also, be sure to make new tapes periodically, especially once you've lost the weight. As you progress with your weight loss, different issues or events may become problems. Changing the tapes from time to time keeps them up-to-date with your concerns and keeps you from getting bored.

Even after you've lost your weight, don't stop listening to your tapes. You don't have to listen every day, but don't cut them out completely. The biggest threat to your weight control is to get cocky and think you're cured. Thin is a lifestyle, not some arbitrary number on a scale. Remember, you lose the weight, you don't lose the problem.

I remember one client who had lost almost 90 pounds when he dropped out of sight for nearly a year. One day he reappeared at my office—with most of the weight regained. He'd gotten out of the habit of listening to the tapes. It was only when he attended his nephew's wedding and overheard a neighbor asking his wife, "What happened to him? He used to look so good!" that he realized how far he had fallen and how much the tapes helped to reinforce his food control.

You may find your tapes to be the strongest weapon you have in your weight-loss arsenal, a frontline defense in the battle for control over your own body. Nowhere is that battle more obvious, more physically palpable, than in the midst of an all-out, full-fledged, stomach-tingling craving. I grant you that many of the battles fought with Food Control Training are won on a psychological level, a level often overlooked by run-of-the-mill diet plans. But you can't ignore the physical—anyone who's ever felt the urges brought on by food knows that the old joke about the pregnant woman making her husband go out in the middle of the night in search of pickles and mint chocolate chip ice cream is no joke. It is a painful reminder of how out of control we can feel, and how diligent and protective of ourselves we must be at all hours of the day or night. Luckily, your food control cassette is just one of many surefire ways you can quell those cravings, wherever and whenever they strike.

STEP FIVE
CONQUER CRAVINGS

Let appetite obey reason.
CICERO

Unlike deprivation, which can creep up and catch you un-awares, cravings arrive with all the subtlety of a Mack truck. You pass a bakery and catch a whiff of the fresh baked bread and suddenly you just *have* to buy a loaf! Or you hear those Good Humor bells or the Mister Softee tune and *pow!*—just as quickly as if someone punched you in the gut or knocked the wind out of you, you feel you can't live without a toasted almond bar or a cone with sprinkles. These "food flashes"—like waves at the beach—can hit anyone. But they don't have to knock you down. Because no matter how vivid the flash, no matter how intense your recall, no matter how powerful the pull, a craving is only a *feeling!* It is not a command!

More importantly, a craving is a feeling that will *pass*—quickly. In fact, research has shown that the average food craving tends to last a mere four to twelve minutes. That's right—four to twelve *minutes!* Not hours, not days, not the eternity it may seem to you at the time. Minutes. In the time it takes to brush your teeth, listen to three songs on the radio, or vacuum your living room rug, the craving will be gone—just like that.

The key, of course, is riding out that crucial four to twelve minutes.

Don't worry, it can be done. Perhaps you've never realized this is a process that you have control over and can stop. It simply doesn't render you powerless, like demonic possession. Demystify it. In fact, once you accept that even the most powerful food craving is only a passing fancy, it's possible to develop the skills you need to sail past food cravings and emerge triumphant—and thin! The trick is being prepared for cravings through proper planning. By developing your own system of Rehearsals, Diversions, Substitutions, and Reality Checks, you can master the fifth step of Food Control Training.

Planning Is Stronger Than Willpower

I've lost count of the number of times I've heard the phrase "I don't have the willpower to resist" when it comes to food cravings. This is an understandable misconception. But it's a misconception nonetheless. Willpower is not some limited, predestined characteristic like the color of your eyes or your height. Willpower is a muscle—and like all muscles it can be strengthened and toned over time. Even more important, from a food control perspective, is the fact that you don't need to rely on *willpower* to conquer cravings—you need a *plan*. More people fail on weight programs because of a lack of planning rather than a lack of willpower. So if you thought you could never succeed because of lack of willpower, this chapter is particularly important for you.

Although cravings strike hard and fast, they rarely come completely out of the blue. They are usually prompted by some external stimulus—for example, the smell of a bakery or pizzeria, the sound of an ice cream truck, or the sight of a candy dish. So even if you can't predict cravings, you can predict the food situations that are likely to prompt cravings. And luckily, since so many of life's situations are predictable, you can *plan* for them. It may never have dawned on you in your entire life that you can actually rehearse your response to them in advance. You can determine how you will act in those situations so that you can keep the occasional food craving from turning into a disaster.

Social situations and events are danger zones for even the most conscientious individual. At parties and other social occasions you are most likely to be faced with the double whammy of trigger foods jutting out in plain sight and well-meaning hosts pressing you to "Please, try some!" That's why you need to be an expert in *defensive eating*.

Defensive eating allows you to prepare yourself for these situations in advance and still enjoy social events without seeming rude or falling prey to your triggers. Here are a few basic rules.

Rule 1: *Never Eat When You're Hungry!* When you were young, you were probably taught to eat when you were hungry. From a control point of view, that lesson doesn't work. Because if you eat when you are hungry, you end up thinking with your taste buds. And when you don't think with your head, you eat impulsively, you eat too much, and you eat too quickly.

Going to a food event on an empty stomach is hazardous to your waistline. *If you arrive empty, you will leave full.* So take measures to curb your appetite. Eat a light meal or a healthy snack beforehand. Drink a glass of chilled tomato juice—some of my most successful clients find it to be a filling and excellent appetite suppressant.

STRESS DON'T EAT MORE; THEY PICK MORE ✧ MORE PEOPLE HAVE

Rule 2: *Don't Be a Food Surveyor!* Remember the old saying "Out of sight, out of mind?" It's certainly true of food. Humans are *visual eaters.* The process of craving begins not with the mouth, but with the eyes. "Oh, it looks so good," you say to yourself, sending out an invitation to cravings in bold embossed letters that read "Come and get me!"

When you arrive at a party, don't scan the room for baskets of chips, cheese and crackers, or guacamole. Instead, take defensive measures to *avoid your triggers.* If you have a problem with hors d'oeuvres, stand by the bar; if your problem is sweets, don't sit by the dessert table; if it's chips, don't stand poised over the coffee table where the basket is placed.

Rule 3: *Don't Negotiate with Food!* Many people, when faced with their old trigger foods, become self-hypnotists. They gaze longingly at the food and actually start negotiating with it. When at a restaurant, faced with the bread basket full of hot rolls, they find themselves thinking, "Oh, you look so good . . . I'll just break off the crust . . . maybe just one." Not only is this a dangerous throwback to the foodie mind-set, it's also rude. Even at the most boring of parties there are better conversationalists to be found than a chocolate raspberry torte. So don't enter into conversations and negotiations with food. Instead, converse with the people around you.

Rule 4: *Conversationally Commit!* A few years ago, one of my clients let me in on her secret weapon for conquering cravings in social situations. Whenever she was at an event where her trigger foods were in evidence, she made a point of mentioning to at least one person that she had sworn off that food or foods. Sometimes that would prompt an entire conversation about weight loss and Food Control Training, sometimes it was simply passed over. But whatever the situation, my client found that once she had conversationally committed herself to abstaining from the food, she was much less inclined to pick.

With a few well-placed words, you too can use your ego as the ultimate brake to save you from your eyes, fingers, and mouth. After all, once you've told someone "Those cookies look great, but I've sworn off them," you aren't likely to let yourself be caught later wolfing them down. This technique is particularly helpful when you are continually around food in your home or office.

Rule 5: *Never Say "Diet"!* When food is being forced upon you by an overeager host, saying you're dieting sometimes can backfire, encouraging a person to say things like "Go back on your diet tomorrow." In these situations, it's best to give a medical reason—"I'm allergic to chocolate" or "My doctor wants me to watch my cholesterol level" or "It's allergy season. I don't drink when I'm on antihistamines"—and you'll usually be left alone. Once you give a medical explanation, the food pushers of this world are disarmed. And don't be concerned about lying, because you're not—it is perfectly honest to say you're allergic to that food for, indeed, when you eat it, you break out in fat.

Rule 6: *Don't Skip Meals—Have Snacks!* You should never go too long without eating a meal. You can prevent cravings from developing (or cut off their power) simply by making sure you don't go hungry. That means being careful not to skip meals or go too long between meals without a snack. Many of my clients note that they have cravings for cakes or candies in the late afternoon. Many who have had long-term problems with flour products or sweets also find that if they skip a meal they don't get hungry for *real* food but rather get "cravey" for these flour products and snacks. In both these cases, the feeling stems from diminishing blood sugar. So make friends with the feeling, and realize your body is simply reminding you it needs to eat.

Rule 7: *Have the Right Food Available!* I'm amazed by how many people get into problems with food simply because of the availability of junk food. Many people—particularly women with the dual responsibility of looking after children and a full-time career—have losses of control when they grab the unhealthy snacks they have around the house for children or other members of their household. You cannot expect to succeed in controlling your weight if you don't have the foods that will help you the most. So make sure you stock your cabinets and refrigerator with the right foods. If you don't have the right foods around, you'll end up wearing the wrong ones.

Rehearsals

Most of us have had moments when we've mentally rehearsed for an event. But did you know that those mental rehearsals actually work? Research on people as diverse as Olympic athletes and corporate executives has shown that people who imagine themselves being successful at a task are more likely to be successful at that task. Simply put, the more you see yourself succeeding, the more likely you are to succeed.

The key, however, is not just *hoping* for a positive outcome, but picturing one that is brought about *by your own efforts*. It's not enough to imagine that the tester at the department of motor vehicles passes you because he likes the color of your eyes. You have to see yourself successfully completing the tasks and actually earning the driver's license. You need to rehearse the skills that will bring you to the desired outcome.

So don't wait until the party is at hand to use the Seven Rules to trigger survival. Practice them in advance. After all, you know what you are likely to see before you go into a restaurant, a wedding reception, or a party at a friend's house. You can anticipate what you will be facing, and when, where, and how you will need to apply the Seven Rules. Just as an actor rehearses a new role, you can rehearse new behaviors to replace the old eating patterns and food dialogues that have become bad habits.

The first step is to stop and think: What situation are you about to enter? Estimate the types and the amounts of food that will be served, and decide what and how much you will choose to eat. Are you having dinner at the home of Great-Aunt Sally, who is always eagerly pushing seconds and thirds onto your plate without even asking? Is it a business engagement, peopled with certain colleagues from work who make you nervous? Consider who is likely to be at the event and how you are likely to react to them. Plan some of the topics you might enjoy discussing and those you might wish to avoid. Make a mental movie of the upcoming event, with yourself as the star—chatting with friends, politely declining foods you should avoid while enjoying those that are not your triggers. Prepare yourself to meet the event not with dread, but with anticipation and pleasure.

Much like Cognitive Switching, this "moviemaking" reorganizes the thoughts you have about food. Only instead of rewriting dialogue, you create scenes in your mind like images on a reel of film. If a picture is worth a thousand words, then using images from your mind will be incredibly powerful in your fight against cravings.

Diversion

Not all cravings strike in social situations. In fact, most people fall prey to cravings right in their own homes, when they are feeling stressed, sad, or just plain bored. In the comfort and privacy of your home it is deceptively easy to say "just this once" and go for a cookie, pretzel, or ice cream when a craving comes calling. On these occasions the best thing you can do is *take a fifteen-minute cooldown.*

Sometimes the most powerful way to beat a craving is not to fight it, but to divert it. If you can take your focus off the craving for fifteen minutes or so, you'll often find that the craving is gone by the end of the cooldown period. Cravings are like waves; they come in quickly and dissipate just as fast. Isn't thin worth the fifteen minutes it will take for the wave to pass? Remember how long you've dreamed about being thin—what's the big deal about riding out a few minutes?

Unlike social craving attacks, which are usually triggered by some external stimulus, at-home cravings are often triggered by emotions or moods: An argument with a spouse, frustration over a malfunctioning appliance, screaming children, and even the midafternoon old doldrums can send anyone into the kitchen. Overcoming that impulse means having alternatives ready and waiting at your fingertips. You need diversions and you need them fast.

Cravings are like fires; to get out unsinged you have to know your emergency exits before the flames are licking at your heels. For cravings, the "emergency exits" are alternative activities that can divert your mind during the crucial fifteen minutes of your cooldown.

The time to plan your emergency exits is now, when you are not in the grip of a craving. Get an index card or piece of paper, title it "Things to Do Instead of Eating," and list several nonfood activities that you can do when a craving strikes. Go for things that will make you feel better and stronger about yourself. Although your list should be as individual as you are, there are a few basic "emergency exits" that everyone should include.

Exit 1: *The Garbage Pail.* If a particular food is calling to you, the first and best defense is to get rid of it. Sometimes, of course, if the food is not yours or the particular situation is unavoidable, this method is impossible. That's when you search for . . .

Exit 2: *The 911 Friend.* The human mind cannot focus on two things simultaneously. You can't focus on a food craving when you're on the phone with a pal. Human emotions and problems require human solutions. Whenever you turn to food for emotional support, you miss out on a chance for human contact. Don't let food occupy a place in your life that should be held by a friend. Find the person or persons in your life who can be a support in times of stress, someone who understands you, perhaps someone who can always make you laugh or feel better about life. Keep their numbers handy. And *call them!* Too often, friends or loved ones say things like "If there's anything I can do . . ." and we never take them up on it. You don't have to make it a therapy session. You don't even have to tell them why you called. Just four or five minutes of pleasant conversation can be as effective and as quickly satisfying as finishing off a box of Pepperidge Farm cookies. Close personal relation-ships enhance every aspect of your life and make it possi-ble to endure the ups and downs of life with far less physi-cal and emotional trauma (as well as far fewer pounds).

Exit 3: *Stress Busters.* Frustration and anger are powerful triggers of self-destructive and uncontrolled eating. If you are a person who eats to relieve stress and frustration, it's time to find some alternative stress busters. Indulge your-self a bit. Buy yourself a dartboard and the next time you're frustrated, throw darts—hard! Designate a pillow as your punching bag. Name it after your boss, if that will help. Start saving old newspapers for recycling and tear them to shreds when you're angry. If simply having something in your hands seems to help, take up needlepoint or knitting or get yourself some sort of tactile toy and keep it around the house. Special stress-busting paraphernalia can be found at specialty stores. Not that it has to get that high-tech: One of my clients has an index card that lists a Slinky, and another will never go anywhere without his Silly Putty.

Exit 4: *Nonfood Rewards.* Food isn't the only rewarding thing in the universe, although that may be hard to remem-ber when you're in the midst of a craving attack. So take the time to list some of the other things in your life that give you pleasure and that can be done in fifteen minutes. Is there a particular song or piece of music that always lifts your spirits? Write it down and note where you keep it. (When you need immediate gratification, you won't have the time or patience to root through your old albums.) How about starting that great book waiting on the shelf? Even a computer game can really psych you up and keep you from noshing. Do long, hot baths make you feel pampered and relaxed? Hit the tub! Does playing with your dog make you feel like a kid again? Take Spot to the park! Let your mind roam free over every aspect of your life to come up with as many sources of nonfood enjoyment as possible.

Exit 5: *Tend to Unfinished Business.* Almost everyone I know has some sort of "to do" list—odds and ends in life that they are always meaning to get around to but somehow never quite do. The fifteen-minute cooldown is a great time to finally get around to some of the projects that have been falling by the wayside, and you can also enjoy a sense of accomplishment as you cross off each completed task. For example, what about that crossword puzzle you started last Sunday? Or that letter you wanted to write your old college roommate? Or the closets that need cleaning out? Or all those back issues of your favorite magazine that you never had time to read?

Exit 6: *Listen to Your Tapes!* That's right, don't forget your tapes, the perfect antidote to almost any craving and the perfect complement to almost any alternate activity. What better way to drown out the voice of your foodie cravings than with your own new dialogue?

Your tapes, that old Simon & Garfunkel album, a chat on the phone, a handful of Silly Putty—silly sounding or not, these are proven techniques that work. By taking the time to look forward and come up with a list of alternatives, weapons that you can use in your battle for thin, the battle itself, when it comes, will seem much more bearable and the war will seem much more winnable.

THE DIET DOCTOR MEETS HIS MATCH

Occasionally, when one of my clients is feeling particularly pressed by cravings for an old favorite food, he or she will say to me, "You don't understand what it's like! You've never had this problem." And I reply that I *do* understand what it is like because I *do* have this problem!

My particular weakness is pizza. It wasn't a problem when I lived in an area where pizza parlors were few and far between. But when I moved into Manhattan I found myself surrounded by excellent pizzerias, many open at all hours. It wasn't long before I was eating pizza several times a day—and seeing the effects.

So I practiced what I preached. Since I couldn't seem to moderate my pizza eating, I eliminated it. After a few months of adjustment, I found it was much easier not to have pizza at all than to try and have it once in a while. But that doesn't mean I don't still have occasional cravings.

I particularly recall one weekend afternoon when I was getting into the elevator, and one of my neighbors came in carrying two boxes of hot, fresh-from-the-oven pizza. As the elevator rose, the smell of crisp crust, sweet tomato sauce, and melted cheese permeated the small space. I found myself glancing at the boxes and remembering how good a fresh slice of pizza could taste. And in almost the same moment I remembered my tightening waistband and that the aroma is really the smell of fat.

I reminded myself that the smell of pizza, and the craving I was feeling, would only be with me for the brief space of the elevator ride. I told myself that as much as I might want a slice of pizza *at that instant*, the moment would pass, and I wanted to be healthy and in control far more. When I said good-bye to my neighbor as he got off at his floor, I was able to continue to my floor without obsessing about pizza or feeling deprived.

That incident was a vivid reminder to me of how tenacious food preferences and cravings can be. Although our minds may change, our taste buds do not. But over time the pull of trigger foods diminishes, and it becomes easier and easier to turn aside when faced with them.

Substitution

Food cravings aren't all in your mind. You crave foods because your body "remembers" the physiological effect the food had when you consumed it in the past. In fact, research has shown that the foods we perceive as enjoyable or rewarding actually activate the same "reward pathways" in the brain that are triggered by certain drugs of abuse—like cocaine. When you experience a "food flash," you are really experiencing a milder form of the drug cravings that afflict recovering addicts.

That's why the smell of food is often all it takes to get you feeling all cravey and distracted. Haven't you on occasion walked past a bakery or entered a friend's kitchen and suddenly the aroma of delicious foods hits you, leaving you tempted? Face it, the smell of food can make you feel hungry as much as the sight of food can. That's a biological fact we're stuck with. The solution is to remind yourself, "That's the aroma of fat cells I don't need."

Luckily, there are other things besides drugs, food, and smells that can activate the reward pathways of your brain. In fact, you can start many of the same internal reactions through exercise, meditation, and—believe it or not—laughter.

Exercise. Exercise, even moderate exercise, can serve as a tremendous antianxiety agent. Research has proven that people who exercise have an enhanced sense of control over their bodies and their lives. Even better, the most recent research indicates that you don't have to run like Flo-Jo or be as much of a hunk as Arnold Schwarzenegger in order to obtain these benefits. The old proviso of at least thirty minutes of exercise three times a week is being modified—shorter bouts of exercise are just as effective. That means a little bit of physical activity for merely ten minutes at a stretch a few times a day is just as effective as the traditional thirty-minute routine. It would seem as if this new research was tailor-made to fit the time needed to overcome the average craving.

Meditation. Whether it is Transcendental or any other kind of meditation, it has been shown to induce a biological state that is the exact opposite of that of stress. Dr. Dean Ornish calls meditation "food for your soul. It satiates the hunger that is not satisfied by food alone. And when your soul is fed, you have less need to overeat. When you directly experience the fullness of life, then you have less need to attempt to fill the void with food."

Lighten Up. Don't take yourself and your weight-loss efforts so seriously that you become grim about it. Laughter lifts depression, soothes anger, and relieves anxiety. Many of my clients keep on hand a videotape of a favorite old comedy or sitcom episode, something that just makes them laugh out loud. You can't laugh and eat at the same time. Humor kills food cravings.

Exercise, meditation, and laughter are three nonfood alternatives that are not only healthy and fun, they give you the scientific edge. With these three substitutions you are not only protecting yourself from the craving, you are changing the underlying chemistry that leads to craving, preventing later attacks.

Reality Checks
Cravings tend to resurrect many of the old foodie messages you want to avoid. Listening to your tapes can help counter

those old messages, but sometimes more aggressive measures are needed. To help reinforce your new food control awareness, I recommend that you develop a few "reality checks" to help you keep things in perspective.

Perhaps the most effective reality check is the simplest: Stick a photo of yourself at your highest weight on the refrigerator. A picture can save a thousand calories. When faced with such a graphic reminder of what going for a trigger food can do to you, it is considerably easier to steer clear of the cabinet or refrigerator.

Another way to attack cravings is to try visualizing other, more long-term negative consequences of out-of-control eating. Just as smokers have heard about black lungs, cancer, emphysema, and heart attacks, most overweight individuals have heard stories of atherosclerosis, heart disease, diabetes, lethargy, and shortened life span. More often than not, we try to push those thoughts out of our minds. It's time to pull those stories out from the storage depot of the mind and into the light. Start really considering those cautions you read in the health columns of magazines and newspapers. Dust off those images of plaque-filled arteries and obesity-induced diabetes. Take a few minutes a day to consider what might happen if your weight continues to increase or ask yourself, is it worth wearing a larger size? You may not experience a sudden miraculous conversion to the world of thin, but you may start feeling a little less seduced by some of those triggers.

Several years ago, researchers at the Institute for Behavior Therapy applied a similar plan of attack to nicotine cravings. Smokers were asked to take ten to fifteen minutes a day to connect a powerful negative image with smoking and concentrate on it. For example, one man pictured himself in the doctor's office hearing the doctor say, "You have emphysema." He would then imagine mourners at his gravesite and his children alongside the coffin, crying, "Why didn't you stop, Daddy?"

If nothing else has worked and you find yourself particularly responsive to aversive stimuli, you can use similar techniques to help conquer food cravings. Imagine the same doctor scene; just change the word *emphysema* to *atherosclerosis* or the phrase "you've developed diabetes." If you want a less dramatic but still disarming image, picture yourself getting up to go to work that morning, opening the closet, starting to get dressed—and then discovering that none of your clothes fit.

Ten to fifteen minutes won't take too much time from your schedule, so try this exercise every day. Perhaps take the first few minutes of your train ride, your eyes closed, not thinking about the day ahead or the other commuters jostling around you, just your image. If you drive to work, call up the image each time you're stopped at a traffic light. Add up all those times waiting for the light to turn green and you've certainly got fifteen minutes of concentration time at your disposal. Or use the time when stuck in that daily traffic jam on the freeway. By exerting a minimum of effort on a consistent basis, you will slowly contribute to your new way of thinking about food.

Whatever reality check you use, keep in mind that *you* are the one using it—it doesn't have to make sense to anyone but you. Some people like to utilize what I call Aversion Therapy 101: They put a picture of a pig on their refrigerator door, for instance. Many find this sort of gimmick humiliating and if it strikes you as such, then I don't advise it. Humiliation is not a key to weight control. But a sense of humor and a realistic perspective are, so if it makes you chuckle and reminds you of your goals, go for a photo of Miss Piggy.

I discovered the surprising power of the Aversion Therapy approach several years ago when one of my clients gave me a rather unusual present. He arrived for a scheduled session bearing a large, yellowish-white, gelatinous-looking mound of plastic "fat."

"Here you go, Dr. Gullo!" he said cheerfully. "The ultimate aversion therapy! Five pounds of ugly fat!"

He was right, it *was* ugly. Revolting, in fact. And though I kept it on my desk throughout our session, I must admit I had every intention of getting it safely out of sight as soon as he left.

But I did not have time to act on my intention, and when my next client arrived she found herself seated eye to eye with a rather disgusting shiny mound of *faux* fat. And she loved it!

"This is *great!*" she exclaimed, picking it up like a football and examining its texture. "It's so gross! If I had this on my kitchen counter, I'd never pick again. Where can I get one?"

Needless to say, the "5 pounds of ugly fat" continues to hold a place of honor on my desk, except on the rare occasion when I have to eat lunch in the office.

Putting It to Work

The best example of conquering cravings that I have ever encountered is the story of a client named Linda. At the time Linda became my client, she was in the midst of a messy and complicated divorce proceeding. For a variety of legal reasons, her husband was still living in the large apartment they had shared since they were first married and they were frequently at home at the same time. Linda's youngest daughter (who was away at college) was very angry about the divorce; her visits home were always tense and often degenerated into tearful fights with Linda.

One rainy winter afternoon, I received a distraught phone call from Linda. Both her husband and her daughter were home, neither wanted to go out because of the rain, and several small blowups had occurred already. Stressed, angry, and trapped with two of the most antagonistic people in her life, Linda was "eating everything in sight." What should she do?

First, I asked Linda exactly what she was eating. She reeled off a list: "Cookies, sesame crackers, potato chips, red grapes—oh, just *everything!*" she said despondently.

"No, you're not eating 'just everything,' " I replied, "you're eating very specific things. Stop for a minute. Think. How does this fit in with your usual pattern?"

Linda has always been a Food Therapist, but she is also a Picker. She never cooks a meal or binges when she's upset. Like almost all stress eaters, Linda doesn't stop and make a lasagna when she's stressed, she goes immediately for finger foods, particularly crunchy ones. She stands at the counter eating chips or randomly pulling finger foods out of the refrigerator. Although she knew that both her husband and daughter would be home that weekend, she had not taken any precautions. She had left the refrigerator and cupboards stocked with precisely the types of foods she would turn to when stress overwhelmed her and had done nothing to ensure that she would be able to get away from her family if necessary.

Within minutes of our conversation, Linda had thrown out the foods she was picking on. Several weeks later, at one of our regular meetings, Linda told me of a very different weekend with her husband and daughter. This time, she planned in advance. She stopped buying the foods she might be prompted to abuse in times of stress and did an inventory of the refrigerator and cupboards the day before her daughter came home. She made a point of scheduling several social events for herself during the weekend so she would not feel trapped. Not surprisingly, the weekend went very well for all concerned. As Linda put it, "I can't control my husband and I can't control my daughter, but I can control what I eat and why. Somehow just knowing that made it a little easier to deal with."

Linda's story incorporates many of the most critical elements of conquering cravings. First and foremost, when a craving hits, you must stop and see the moment for what it is. It's just a moment, just a short period of time in your day, something you can deal with, but something you must deal with right away.

Second, get away from the food. Walk out of the kitchen, out of the living room, out of the office. And take several long, deep breaths.

Now you're ready to start dealing effectively with the event. Give your 911 Friend a call.

If your 911 Friend is unavailable, grab your index card (taking a quick glimpse at that photo of you at your highest weight, if it's within view) and start going down your list. Where are you, how much time do you have, and what things on the list can you do *right now* to occupy your time for the next fifteen minutes or so? Is music on your list? Grab that favorite record and play it. Mr. Bubble handy? Get in the tub! Is it a nice day out? Take a stroll around the block. Remember, this time is for you, a special recuperative period that you should not feel guilty about taking. After all, it's only fifteen minutes. And once that fifteen minutes is past and you have enjoyed your bath, your walk, your dartboard, or your meditation, you will find that the craving has subsided.

Of course, there will be times when, despite all your good intentions, despite listening faithfully to your tapes, despite your awareness of the cultural programming that affects us all, you will still succumb to the old ways. The cravings will come. And despite all your valiant efforts, there is bound to be one that will catch you by surprise and throw you off balance.

None of us are made of steel. It happens to the winners of Food Control Training just like everyone else. But Food Control Training allows for those mistakes and gives you some room to be human and fallible. In the next chapter, I will discuss the various ways in which you can turn these blunders to your advantage.

STEP SIX
CONTAINMENT

To err is human.
ALEXANDER POPE

People make mistakes. They always have and they always will. If they didn't, pencils wouldn't need erasers. Do you know anyone who has mastered a skill without making a single error? Mistakes are an inevitable part of life and an inevitable part of food control, because, unlike dieting, food control is a life management skill. It doesn't end on the fateful day you reach your target weight.

Thin is a skill, and like any skill—from tennis to piloting a 747—it takes practice. If you stop concentrating and paying attention to good form, occasional missteps will happen, just as they do in any sport. Tennis players double-fault. Golfers slice. Healthy, slender people eat entire bags of pretzels.

The ability to contain these mistakes—to prevent minor slips from turning into major landslides—is the final and most important of the survival steps that set the winners at weight loss apart from most dieters. So many people have gone to almost every weight program in existence without ever learning this central skill. Containment is the culmination of all the lessons of Food Control Training. It is the skill that incorporates everything you've learned about your relationship with food and the nature of control. Once you've mastered this strategy, you will have truly mastered your control problem with food.

Keep It in Perspective!

Never say "I blew it." It undermines your containment skills like no other phrase or thought. The best diet counselors, diet books, and diet plans all know that a far better response to an occasional slipup—no matter how extreme—is to say nothing, do nothing.

That's right—nothing! Don't berate yourself for your failure. Don't give up and eat everything else in sight. Don't try to make up for it by starving yourself later. Don't try to work off the extra calories by exercising obsessively.

In fact, the only realistic way to handle an occasional dietary slip is to acknowledge your mistake, pick yourself up, and get on with your life. You can't turn back the hands of time. You can't make the calories go away. There's no sense in punishing yourself or trying to make up for your brief slip. That's the road to paranoia, despair, and eating disorders. It's normal to feel some guilt when you've broken a commitment to yourself but feeling guilty and beating yourself up won't burn up any calories. Only stopping the behavior and moving on will remedy the slip.

Think about it. Do you know anyone who has mastered a skill without making an error? Even the greatest hitters in baseball's Hall of Fame never batted a thousand.

Most people, however, aren't that forgiving when it comes to their own life. They react to the occasional poor food choice (and remember, you always have a choice) as if it signaled the end of the world. They assume that because they blew it once, they've lost control forever and they use that single slip as an excuse for going back to all their old patterns. "What the heck?" they say. "I pigged out at lunch, so today is shot—I might as well order up that deadly dessert."

But the defeatist "I blew it and I have to punish myself to make up for it" approach to slips is just another way of turning control of your life over to food.

If you occasionally slip up in the practice of food control, don't go into a tailspin of despair and reproach. Keep your perspective. You didn't completely surrender your free will just because you made one poor food choice. You can and will do better in the future. And the future starts now.

Beware the "Tomorrow" Trap

"I'll start again tomorrow." How many times have you said that in the past? And how many times did tomorrow remain just one day away—when you'd be feeling a little better, a little more motivated, a little less pressured or depressed? That's the funny thing about "tomorrow" and food control—it never seems to come.

"Tomorrowisms" are one of the main reasons people fail, if only momentarily, at their weight-loss efforts. Instead of getting on with the business of life, tomorrow people spend their time negotiating with food, coming up with new and ever-more-creative rationalizations for putting control off until the next day. With just four little words—"I'll start again tomorrow"—they fling open the doors and invite triggers back into their lives. And once those triggers have gotten a foothold, they aren't going anywhere.

If you slip up, you don't have the option of waiting until tomorrow to take back control. Even if you can't take back your mistake, you can stop yourself from making another one. Every food choice is another opportunity for exercising control and free will or for knuckling under to the old programming.

If you feel yourself succumbing to tomorrowisms, uncertainty and indecisiveness have crept into your life. The technical term I use to describe this is cognitive ambivalence. Simply, you have gotten caught between your old foodie beliefs and your new, healthy belief system. You want to stay thin, but you're being seduced by the old deprivation mind-set.

Tomorrowisms enter your life along with this cognitive ambivalence. They are a compromise maneuver—a way of fooling yourself into believing that you really can indulge yourself "just this once." It's okay, you'll be good again tomorrow, right?

Wrong! If you are honest with yourself, you'll admit that you won't be good tomorrow. If you slip up, you need to "be good" immediately. Not in ten minutes, not in an hour, not tomorrow, now!

Whenever you hear yourself using the "tomorrow" rationale, you know you are in trouble. That pesky little id is getting the upper hand and you are forgetting the hard-learned lessons of your Eating Print. Sometimes, regaining control can be rather simple. In fact, many of my clients have told me that the two most powerful words you can say to yourself to cut short a slip-up are *Stop now!* Using this technique can help you snap out of your forlorn state if you truly listen to those words. And that's not the only way you can prevent such slides into cognitive ambivalence and tomorrowisms.

The Periodic Checkup: Using the New Scale

Every slipup has the potential to be a learning experience. Every temporary loss of control can teach you a little more about what you can or cannot handle, what still triggers taste buds, and what situations you still need to avoid. Slowly but surely, you can use your slips to develop a foolproof map for navigating around your triggers.

But you don't have to wait for a slipup to change your course. Just as a good captain regularly checks his depth gauge to be sure he doesn't run aground, you can periodically sound the level of your food control. This way, you can tell when you are straying into shallow waters.

A scale is not the instrument to use when checking your level of food control. After all, every fat person owns a scale! In Food Control Training, the best measure of control is a simple six-question quiz that I call the New Scale. This quiz reviews some of the basic skills and attitudes you should be maintaining as part of your healthy life of thin. With it, you can track changes in your control skills much as a diabetic tracks her blood sugar or a person with hyper-

---

THE NEW SCALE

Give yourself this quiz about once a week. If you've slipped or found yourself falling into the old foodie belief systems, admit it. Evaluate when, where, and why it occurred. See if there are any cues you can be alert to in the future to prevent similar problems from occurring.

1. Have I had (or thought of having) any of my trigger foods or gotten into my trigger situations?
2. Have I lost control of or abused any of my nontrigger foods?
3. Have I negotiated with food?
4. Have I thought like a fat person, glorifying food?
5. Have I maintained finger control?
6. Have I bought any of my trigger foods or kept them in the house?

---

tension monitors his blood pressure. With regular use, it can alert you to the areas in which you may still be a little weak and therefore vulnerable to slipups.

For most successful dieters, cognitive ambivalence and tomorrowisms take a while to surface. You may go for months without a hint of doubt, untroubled by temptation. When cognitive ambivalence does make an appearance, it can be a pretty nasty surprise. "Why is this happening now?" you may ask. "What am I doing wrong?"

More than likely, you're not doing anything wrong. You've just reached one of the later—and more problematic—stages of dieting.

The Six Stages of Dieting

Weight loss, like everything else in life, occurs in stages, over time. Each stage is marked by very different emotions and levels of motivation. To maintain your weight—and control over food—you need to be aware of where you are in these stages, and—if necessary—take steps to bolster your flagging motivation and confidence.

Stage 1: *Pain and Desperation.* Often characterized by very strong, very negative feelings. You may feel disgusted with yourself for your lack of control or hate to look at yourself in the mirror. Although this is often the stage that propels overweight people into treatment, it can also become a black hole, in which the motivation to change is overwhelmed by a sense of futility and self-loathing.

Stage 2: *Action.* The point at which you make the crucial move of getting into some sort of weight program or putting yourself on a diet. You're fed up with being fed up. Instead of hating yourself or fantasizing about being thin, you decide to take matters into your own hands and actually lose the weight. Motivation and commitment are typically very high.

Stage 3: *Structure.* You start applying the principles of the weight program to your day-to-day life. You set up a schedule for yourself, plan what to eat, and eliminate some foods from your diet. Although motivation and commitment are high during this stage, they can easily be undermined by the deprivation mind-set if some kind of Cognitive Switching isn't begun.

Stage 4: *Recognition.* The turning point, second only to maintenance as the stage most likely to prompt a relapse. You are beginning to see results. Your clothes feel looser, you see more definition in your face, you have more stamina and endurance. These rewards can either work for or against you. If you've been making the necessary cognitive switches, you understand that you may be losing the weight but you have not lost the problem. Just because the pounds come off doesn't change your taste buds or your vulnerability to your trigger foods. Ideally, recognition will reinforce your determination to maintain control and make it increasingly easy to say no to your triggers. If you have not made the cognitive switch, however, this stage may lead to the Great Lie. You may believe that because you've lost a few pounds you've also lost your control problems with certain foods. Instead of avoiding triggers, you may try to reward yourself with "just a little," setting off on the slippery slope that is ruled by the F/Q Principle. If that occurs, you will find yourself at a plateau, since the cheating puts a stop on your weight loss or even puts the pounds back on as your motivation falters. Call it "diet burnout" or whatever you want, but at this point it's absolutely critical to force your motivation, since you may find yourself thinking, "I don't feel like doing this anymore."

Stage 5: *Success.* Success is exactly that. You've reached your weight goal! Every time you look in the mirror you feel a little thrill of pleasure. The intense satisfaction of having achieved your treasured goal convinces you that you'll never go back to the old ways again. Motivation and commitment are high.

Stage 6: *Maintenance.* The most high-risk stage of any weight-control effort. It comes as the rush of success starts to wear off. You've gotten used to seeing your new self in the mirror. Your friends are no longer amazed at your appearance. The honeymoon is over and you are getting down to the business of living thin.

Maintenance is the stage where cognitive ambivalence, tomorrowisms, and the Great Lie are most likely to rear their ugly heads. The pain and desperation of Stage 1 seem a million miles away. Instead of remembering the misery you felt when you were the fattest person at your niece's wedding, you remember the texture and taste of the chocolate raspberry wedding cake. Instead of recalling how embarrassed you felt when you couldn't join your daughter in the sack race at the company picnic, you remember licking barbecue sauce off your fingers as you ate a rack of spareribs.

Now, more than ever, you need to make use of your tapes, your Cognitive Switching, and the lessons of your Eating Print. Keep pictures of your old, unhappy self around as vivid reminders of what the good old days were really like. Fill your life with the nonfood alternatives dis-

WHAT THEY EAT BEFORE, AFTER, AND IN BETWEEN MEALS THAN FROM

cussed under Step Five and revel in the physical and the healthy foods you now enjoy. Remember, the process, not just a number on a scale or a clothing size, is the destination. And, as always, remember—no matter what the food—thin tastes better!

Preventive Medicine

Sometimes recovering from a mistake requires psychological CPR—you may need to resuscitate your psyche to get the motivation to go forward. The best way to do this is to take one meal at a time, slowly but surely piecing together one small success after another. With each successful food encounter, you will feel your sense of self-mastery grow.

Most food control slips—including the most catastrophic ones—are the result of momentary memory lapses. When most people slip, they have not only forgotten the lessons of their Eating Print, they have forgotten all of the other nonfood options that are available to them—often because they have not been properly exercising those options. Because of this, one of the most effective methods of containment is prevention.

You can prevent momentary indiscretions from becoming monumental disasters by staying involved in activities that bolster your sense of vitality and control without involving food. Go back to the diversions and fifteen-minute cooldown (pages 132–135) for ideas. And remember:

Keep Moving. If you've stopped going to the gym, go back. In addition to improving your health, increasing your resting metabolism, and building muscle mass, exercise generates neurochemicals that lift your spirits and reduce your appetite. The time and sweat you put in at the gym can give you a sense of control of your body even if you're still overweight. And this sense of control will transfer to your eating behavior.

Hook into a Support Network. If you're having trouble going it alone consider joining a weight-control program or self-help group like Overeaters Anonymous. You can gain a lot even from just a few visits. If such organized groups don't appeal to you, why not form a group of your friends who have similar problems? Perhaps get together for a card game instead of a formal meeting that may make everyone feel awkward. It is far more productive for those who share this problem to meet together and discuss it than to keep the feelings bottled up inside.

Get a Buddy. Another option is to form an alliance with one particular friend who is working on weight problems, and at the time of the day when you have the most difficulty, call each other.

Be creative in developing your behavioral strategies for outmaneuvering food. You are always starting with a great advantage. You have the intelligence, the smarts. The food has none.

Coping in the Real World: What to Do When You Have No Choice

The way you can contain the errors in your life need not interfere with your social life nor drain your life of fun. Containment is not a punishment or penance. It is an instructional tool that should make you feel better about yourself, your weight, and your progress with food control.

I don't expect you to live like a hermit. You have to interact with people, go places, and live your life in the real world. That means that there are bound to be times when you will be in situations where there aren't many smart food choices available. You may be at a business lunch, a wedding reception, or a special family gathering where the foods served are—if not your triggers—at least chock-full of calories and fat. These special circumstances require special food control strategies.

If you look to most etiquette books, you will be told that unless you have a life-threatening food allergy, good manners requires that you "take at least a little of every dish that is offered to you, which can be spread out on your plate so that it is barely noticeable that you have not eaten much." However, "it would be wasteful and upsetting if you took a portion and left it untouched."

Of course, this is just the kind of advice that a person with food control problems—particularly a Finisher—absolutely does not need to hear!

So, to enjoy life and maintain control in the real world, take my advice: Politely refuse a portion of *anything* that could make you lose control.

Believe me, your host or hostess will not be insulted if you pass up one particular item on the menu. No one will mind if you skip a roll, the hors d'oeuvres, or a dessert for medical reasons. Remember, you are always telling the truth, because being overweight is a life-threatening illness.

You just need to be selective. It's not as if I'm suggesting you pass up the entrée. If there is a creamy sauce, ask to have it served on the side. If you're like most people, you're likely to have gained your weight from the finger foods (breads, rolls, fatty hors d'oeuvres, cheeses) and desserts at a dinner party than from the main course. It is not at all essential that you eat all of these accessories. Take onto your plate only those foods you feel confident you can control.

If the entrée is rather fattening and you can't escape it or you do have some of your trigger foods at a party, forget about it. Once you leave the party, it's over. Treat it as a single isolated incident and don't waste time blaming yourself or feeling guilty. Remember the truth about your weight: It is not the isolated incident of a dinner party or affair but what you eat on a day-to-day basis that makes you heavy.

Rather than blaming yourself once you get home, look for the patterns of what went wrong. Did you go to the party hungry and so ate compulsively? Could you have brought a gift of a low-fat frozen yogurt dessert to your hostess, thereby subtly providing your own safe dessert? Did you sit in front of the bread basket and not ask for it to be moved— or not move yourself when you could easily have done so? Were you surveying the foods instead of talking to the other guests? Did you go to the event without any dress rehearsal, without a glass of tomato juice, with no preparation whatsoever?

In the end, the ultimate significance of a social slipup is that you now know you must practice your control skills more in party situations. Not everyone at the party ate everything that was offered. Next time, you can be one of them. Next time, you can say, "No, thank you," to the food and say "yes" to being thin.

Mastering the Six Steps

When we were growing up, we read the fairy tales about finding the magical prince or princess and living happily ever after. In the real world, happiness takes work. Life is a process of fielding the curveballs as well as the home runs of life. It is a process of self-mastery, where happiness and disappointment and even despair at times are part of the journey. And the key to this process is *resilience*.

I have seen it work for the winners. They have learned how to bounce back, no matter what the circumstances, no matter what the goof or blunder they committed. It is this resilience that you want to nurture in yourself.

Becoming resilient takes sustained effort, but not nearly as much effort as it takes to live fat. On the day when you find working on control to be the hardest, the most unbearable, or the most unwinnable, remember that there is a world out there reeling from cancer, AIDS, homelessness. And if the most you have to worry about is merely controlling a piece of food, then you have a pretty good deal.

It is not a deal you should exchange for a measly crumb of food. When a piece of food endangers the quality of life itself, when you cannot run and play with the kids because your weight makes you easily winded, when you cannot enjoy a night out on the town with the one you love because you despise the way you look in your clothes, when your doctor has told you that your cholesterol is way too high and that you are a heart attack waiting to happen, when your dissatisfaction with the image you see in the mirror affects how confidently or aggressively you present yourself at work or in the community, when how you look prevents you from meeting people or asking somebody out on a date or just going up to a person and saying "hello," then *there is no choice, there is no contest—that food or foods must go.*

You can eliminate what you cannot control and still enjoy the joys of good food. You can avoid or limit the foods and behaviors that once tripped you up and still feel satisfied after a meal. You can feed the champion within you and keep your motivation burning by mastering the secrets of shopping, preparing, and cooking food that were previously known only to that elusive and lucky 5 percent. The winners have surefire ways of shopping and cooking and I will pass them on to you.

Remember, the key to food control—and weight control—is resilience. So ignore whatever anxieties or lingering doubts you may have and go with the energy and anticipation of your new, healthy, truly thin self. Even if you slip, you'll pick yourself up and move on. Because no slipup—no matter how serious it may seem—is insurmountable. You can take your occasional mistakes, learn from them, and come away even stronger. Don't let a single mistake with a glob of calories undermine all that you have learned and achieved. The slips in life should teach us, not defeat us.

PART THREE

WHAT TO EAT

THE FOOD CONTROL
EATING PLAN

> *I want to be lean, not fat, and no flavor of
> ice cream in the world could ever tempt me
> enough to end up at that ice cream parlor
> dying of shame. None.*
> SUSAN POWTER

The most frequent question asked by my clients is not "How much should I lose?" or even "How long will it take?" It is: "What should I eat?"

Ultimately, the answer is simple: You can eat well, you can eat amply, you can, in fact, eat just about anything—as long as it isn't among your trigger foods. Foods aren't good or bad—they're just collections of chemicals and calories. Foods *become* good or bad when you make them so: when you eat a few foods to the exclusion of all others, when you cannot eat a specific food without losing control, or when you believe that in order to have it all you have to eat it all.

By now you have a clear view of the overall mosaic of your eating history. You understand your Eating Print and you know the cultural, personal, and behavioral patterns that have led you down the road to overweight. And you know that your goal is not just to lose weight, but to *permanently change those patterns*—by changing your mind *and* your eating behaviors.

❖ WHEN YOU CAN'T HAVE EVERYTHING YOU WANT, YOU CAN STILL

The Six Steps of Food Control Training are the key to changing your mind. The Food Control Eating Plan is the key to changing your consumption.

The plan is a simple guide to foods that give you taste, texture, and excellent nutrition without giving you unneeded calories and fat. It is also a guide to the foods that my clients and I have found to be least associated with losses of control.

The plan isn't a diet in the usual sense of the word, i.e., a temporary program of restricted eating that lasts only until you've lost weight. The Food Control Eating Plan is a whole new way of living, one that the winners of weight loss are happy to choose because it frees them from the pounds of fat, losses of control, guilt, and sense of deprivation that once ruled their lives. Most importantly, it frees them from the belief that following a healthy eating plan means missing out on the good foods of life, whether eating out or eating in.

You will use the plan to chart all of your future meals, not just the ones you are eating while trying to lose weight. It will become your new baseline, the norm to which you will return after having an occasional "boxed in" trigger food. It's a healthy norm, a delicious norm, a norm that is supported by the experience of the winners *and* the best of nutritional research. It is, in short, a norm you will feel good about living with.

The Basics

The winners who lose weight and keep it off do far more than strike a healthy balance on their bathroom scales. They also strike a healthy and comfortable balance in their daily diet. They know which foods can give them the flavors, textures, and pleasures of fine dining without undermining their sense of control, and they adapt their eating behaviors to meet any food situation. The Food Control Eating Plan is based on the example of these people. It meets the psychological, nutritional, physiological, and social needs of those with weight problems, and it does it in the context of the real world.

First and foremost, the plan recognizes that people with *weight* problems are, by definition, people with *quantity* problems. If they could have "just a little," they would not be overweight in the first place. I have yet to meet an overweight person who did not have a deep, basic need for generous portions, a need that is reinforced by almost every cultural message we have ever received about food. As several of my clients have said, "It's a lot easier to not have it at all than it is to try and leave half on my plate!"

Rather than deny (or fight) this basic need, the plan is *generous.* It has been designed to meet your need for quantity by emphasizing foods that *can* be eaten in large amounts. In fact, the entire Food Control Eating Plan is based on one guiding premise: *White is light and green is lean!*

White—as in protein sources such as seafood, fish, poultry, low-fat cheeses, and egg-white omelettes—and green—as in green vegetables. These nutrient-rich foods are so naturally low in calories and fat that you can enjoy very generous amounts without fear, particularly when you prepare them according to the guidelines in the next chapter. So think white and green and you will always know what to eat for lunch and dinner.

The plan also recognizes that in our culture people tend to eat their largest amount of calories late in the day, when the body is least efficient at burning those calories. Because starchy pastas and breads are not a good choice for the last meal of the day, the plan emphasizes low-fat protein sources and fiber-rich vegetables that can give the body the thermogenic edge it needs late in the day.

The plan also recognizes that eating is more than just a biological function; it is also a pleasurable social event. The best diet plan is therefore one that not only tastes good but that will also work in the real world of holidays, dinner parties, restaurants, business lunches, and the like. For this reason, the plan is *realistic*. It is based on foods you can find in any supermarket, foods that are found at most dinner parties, foods you can order in any restaurant, and foods that you will actually want to eat.

Finally, because the perfect diet for you can only be designed by you, the Food Control Eating Plan is *flexible*. It can be adjusted to meet the parameters of your Eating Print, your work schedule, your living situation, and any of the other realities of your day-to-day life. On the plan you can adapt to any situation, including occasions when there seems to be no choice. And unlike many weight-loss plans, it recognizes the essential metabolic and hormonal differences between men and women and the effect those differences have on appetite and weight loss.

The White and Green Pyramid Plan

The Food Control Eating Plan is built around four pyramids (see pages 168–169) that indicate the frequency of intake for certain types of foods during weight loss and maintenance for men and women. Vegetables, for example, should always be consumed at least three times a day, in meals and as snacks. However, since not all vegetables are created equal, the chart on page 175 provides information on the recommended number of servings. Charts on pages 176 through 179 contain similar information for the other classes of foods outlined in the pyramids.

The Food Control Pyramids, unlike the USDA's Food Guide Pyramid, are meant specifically for those with weight problems. They have been influenced by the research of scientists such as Dr. Artemis Simopoulos, Drs. Rachael and Richard Heller, and Dr. Shari Lieberman, as well as my own experience with thousands of successful clients. Dr. Lieberman also reviewed my eating plan from a nutritional point of view. The pyramids have been designed to meet both your nutritional needs and your control needs. As a result, they emphasize vegetables, fruits, and low-fat protein far more than grains and grain-based foods. They don't ask you to limit yourself to a tiny portion of pasta or brown rice. They don't require you to compulsively weigh every morsel of food that passes your lips. Instead, they set simple, realistic guidelines for planning your meals and food choices.

These are guidelines, not laws. As you plan your meals and your life of thin, evaluate these guidelines in the light of your own unique Eating Print. Because *control comes before calories!*

Don't include a food in your diet plan if it is a food (or type of food) that you have a long history of abusing. Seemingly benign "low-fat," "lite," and "diet" foods—from oat bran pretzels to microwaved chips to nonfat frozen desserts—can be just as dangerous as their high-fat counterparts if they are among your trigger foods.

Indeed, maintaining food control (and weight loss) may sometimes mean making what some would call the wrong food choices. If you are a carbo craver at a dinner party where the only choices are filet mignon or a pasta dish, the seemingly fattening steak—with all of its saturated fat and

---

calories—is a better choice for you than the seemingly healthy pasta. While the beef may give you more calories and fat *at that single, isolated meal,* it will at least be limited to that meal. It won't trigger old cravings or additional losses of control.

Recently, one of my clients learned this lesson the hard way. She was at a sit-down dinner party where the entrée was roast beef, a delicious but decidedly fat-laden dish. Wanting to avoid the saturated fat in the roast beef, my client decided to fill up on the fresh whole grain bread that was being served.

Unfortunately, this woman is also extremely sensitive to carbohydrates. She was hungry and craving bread within a few hours of the dinner party. By the time I saw her again, about a week later, she had fallen back into many of her old out-of-control eating patterns and had gained back 3 pounds.

No matter what common "nutritional wisdom" may say, control—not calories or even fat—must be the ultimate arbiter when it comes to choosing foods. Whether you are in a restaurant, at a party, or in the supermarket, if a food can't pass the Control Test (see page 43), it should not pass your lips. If you abused it in the past, you will abuse it in the future.

Calorie Units: A New Way to Count Calories

The best way to evaluate a food in terms of its control risk is to think in terms of *calorie units* rather than calories per serving. Many foods that seem perfectly safe and low calorie on the basis of calories per serving become something else altogether when you think of how many servings you will actually *consume.*

Diet cookies, pretzels, and other low-calorie or low-fat snack foods can be very tempting because of optimistic labels that trumpet "only 10 calories per cookie!" But the labels forget that the natural inclination of all humans is not to eat one or two, but to be a Finisher. When was the last time you met someone who could stop at one or two peanuts or a single handful of popcorn? If you have a bag of some snack food, even if it is a small one, you are most likely going to finish the whole thing. So the true calorie content of that food isn't the number of calories in one item or serving, it's the number of calories in one item times the number of units you typically consume.

For example, a popular brand of oat bran pretzels contains no fat, plenty of fiber, and a mere 60 calories per serving (one pretzel). Sounds like a good deal, right? But when was the last time you ate only one pretzel? Most people will eat half a dozen without blinking an eye, and if you're a Picker it's a good bet that you'll finish the entire bag of eighteen pretzels. So for you, that one "low-calorie, nonfat" pretzel really contains 1,080 calories! Not quite such a good deal, is it?

Some Rules of the Road

The first thing to keep in mind before you start a weight-loss program is the importance of consulting a physician who can properly evaluate your physical condition, monitor your progress, and keep you informed about the changes you will see and feel in your body. Once you get the go-ahead from your doctor, then it's time to think about what to eat and what not to eat.

In addition to your own Eating Print and the guidelines of the pyramids and their associated tables, there are sev-

FOOD CONTROL PYRAMIDS: MEN

(For specific servings, see pages 175–179)

Weight Loss

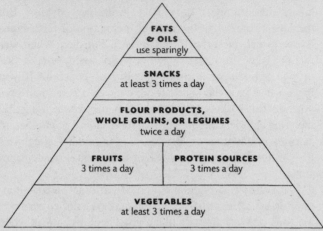

FATS & OILS
use sparingly

SNACKS
at least 3 times a day

FLOUR PRODUCTS, WHOLE GRAINS, OR LEGUMES
twice a day

FRUITS
3 times a day

PROTEIN SOURCES
3 times a day

VEGETABLES
at least 3 times a day

Alcoholic beverages: 3 per week*

Maintenance

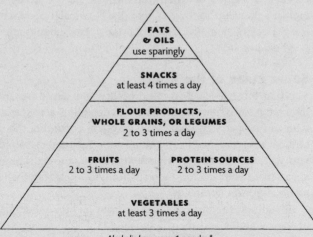

FATS & OILS
use sparingly

SNACKS
at least 4 times a day

FLOUR PRODUCTS, WHOLE GRAINS, OR LEGUMES
2 to 3 times a day

FRUITS
2 to 3 times a day

PROTEIN SOURCES
2 to 3 times a day

VEGETABLES
at least 3 times a day

Alcoholic beverages: 1 per day*

**1 serving = 1 glass of wine *or* 1 beer *or* 1 mixed drink*

FOOD CONTROL PYRAMIDS: WOMEN

(For specific servings, see pages 175–179)

Weight Loss

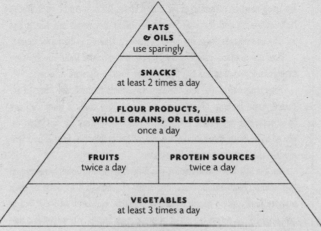

FATS & OILS
use sparingly

SNACKS
at least 2 times a day

FLOUR PRODUCTS, WHOLE GRAINS, OR LEGUMES
once a day

FRUITS
twice a day

PROTEIN SOURCES
twice a day

VEGETABLES
at least 3 times a day

Alcoholic beverages: 2 per week*

Maintenance

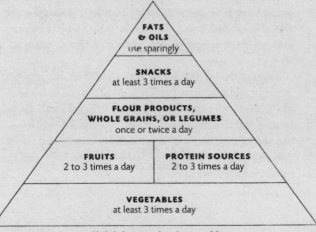

FATS & OILS
use sparingly

SNACKS
at least 3 times a day

FLOUR PRODUCTS, WHOLE GRAINS, OR LEGUMES
once or twice a day

FRUITS
2 to 3 times a day

PROTEIN SOURCES
2 to 3 times a day

VEGETABLES
at least 3 times a day

Alcoholic beverages: 3 to 6 per week*

*1 serving = 1 glass of wine or 1 beer or 1 mixed drink

EATING LESS FAT/GAINING MORE WEIGHT

The good news is: according to the United States Department of Agriculture's National Health and Nutrition Survey (NHANES), Americans are eating less fat. The bad news is: there are more overweight Americans than ever before.

How are so many people getting fat on nonfat foods? Quite simply, even though they're eating less fat, they are also consuming more calories.

For many nutritional scientists and weight-loss professionals, myself included, these findings are no surprise. In fact, they confirm what we have been observing for years. The problem of excess dietary fat has been replaced by a much more insidious problem: the problem of how—and how much—the American people are eating.

We live in a snack food culture, and Americans are increasingly relying on high-calorie, high-carbohydrate, and easily abused snack products as their primary foods. Many people even skip breakfast and lunch entirely, and at around 3:00 P.M. a nonstop buffet of snack foods begins. We are settling into a pattern of constant picking, and the effects are being seen in the nation's expanding waistlines.

It is even possible that the increased number of low- and no-fat foods may be contributing to this nationwide weight gain. Preliminary research on the effect of low-fat foods indicates that, for some people, a low-fat label serves as a cue to eat more, regardless of the number of calories they actually consume.

I have lost count of the number of clients who could not understand how they had gained weight when they were so careful about the fat in their diets. "It doesn't make sense," they say. "I only eat nonfat foods!" But the lessons of the Eating Print will not be denied. If you abused the high-fat version, you *will* abuse the low-fat version (perhaps even more), and you *will* gain weight. "Nonfat" does not mean "not fattening," no matter what advertisers would have you believe.

eral basic rules to keep in mind when choosing foods. These rules will help you pick foods that are both good nutritional investments and low control risks.

1. Choose foods that are as fresh and unprocessed as possible. The more processed a food is, the fewer nutrients it contains and the more dramatic its effect on your blood sugar levels. A canned pear has a lot less flavor, fiber, and nutrients than a fresh one, and whole grains are far more nutritious (and tasty) than refined, bleached, or even enriched flours.

2. Avoid starchy, flour-based foods. Despite the current fad touting pasta (which the dictionary defines as a "flour paste"), breads, and other flour-based products, these foods are anything but nonfattening when consumed by people with control problems. More of my clients have gained weight because of starch than because of fat. There is really no comparison between a supposedly low-fat, low-calorie restaurant entrée such as spaghetti with marinara sauce (1,180 calories/21.2 grams of fat) and an entrée of grilled sole (260 calories/2.75 grams of fat). Besides being lower in fat and calories, the fish has 50 percent more protein and more than twice the calcium of the pasta dish, as well as being an excellent source of heart-healthy omega-3 fatty acids. Perhaps most important, the 55 grams of protein in the sole are far more thermogenic than the 220 grams of carbohydrate in the pasta, so you will burn more of the calories you take in. And unlike pasta—which is likely to set off a cycle of craving in carbohydrate-sensitive people—the fish meal leaves you feeling satisfied for a much longer period of time.

DON'T TAKE THE FIRST LITTLE TASTE, I DON'T BEGIN. I DON'T HAVE ANY

3. Avoid foods that contain more than 25 percent of their calories in fat. This should be the maximum amount you allow yourself. The new food labels very conveniently list the percentage of calories from fat right at the top, so it's easy to tell. Remember, fat builds fat, so the more you eat, the more your body will tuck away into your fat cells. Seafood, fresh vegetables, whole grains, and poultry can give you the healthy fats your body needs.

4. Avoid foods that are served in unlimited quantities. Big bowls of mashed potatoes, rice, and pastas and the kinds of heaping servings seen more and more at family-style restaurants tend to bring out the Finisher in the best of us. Such abundant visions of food are a potent trigger, and the more we see the more we feel compelled to eat. It's rare to go to a restaurant and not feel satisfied with the size of a single serving. But when seconds and thirds are available many people feel that a single serving is completely inadequate and automatically go back for refills. Even when a food is a fairly good nutritional investment (such as brown rice or whole grain pasta), it is sometimes wise to pass in the interest of maintaining control. Avoid serving such foods at home, and when you do, monitor the amount you serve yourself to prevent losses of control.

5. Avoid finger foods. Everyone has a bit of a Picker in them, and finger foods may well be the universal trigger. When in doubt, steer clear of foods that don't require a plate and some utensils. This rule applies to healthy finger foods too, especially finger fruits (like grapes or cherries) or cut-up fruits. Limit your consumption of finger foods to specific, infrequent occurrences, such as popcorn at the movies. Many of my clients enjoy air-popped popcorn at the movies but never have it at home because it could easily become a daily habit. They know that if they have it at home they could easily fall back into a behavior of continual noshing and end up eating far more than just popcorn. When popcorn consumption is limited to the movies, they end up having one small bag every few weeks and the behavior is contained.

6. Diversify. Most of us have incredibly monotonous diets! Despite the fact that we can get almost any fruit, vegetable, meat, or grain at any time of the day or year, we eat the same basic foods day in and day out, year after year. The single best way to keep your diet interesting and nutritionally sound is to keep it varied. When is the last time you ate a fresh mango? Or a grilled sweet potato? Or a seafood kabob? There's an entire universe of foods available to be explored.

7. But don't overdo it. There is a real danger in having too many tempting varieties of foods—even healthy ones—on hand at any given time. I have found, without exception, that *availability creates craving and variety stimulates consumption.* So while it is important to vary your diet and enjoy a wide range of healthy foods, the presence of many different fruits in the house *at the same time* can lead to overconsumption and impede your weight-loss efforts. What you are doing is creating a buffet, and people with weight problems rarely do well at buffets—whether it's a buffet of fruit or one of desserts. It is important to eat a variety of good foods, but don't necessarily bring them all home at the same time.

8. When in doubt, think seafood and fish. After watching the progress of thousands of clients, I believe seafood and fish are the fastest route to weight loss. And with the huge variety of shellfish and freshwater and saltwater catches available, and the seemingly infinite number of ways to prepare them, everyone can find *something* they like.

IT'S NOT JUST CALORIES . . .
KNOW THE CONTROL VALUE OF ANY FOOD

All foods have a calorie value. They also have a Control Value—a rating that shows you which foods pose serious threats to control and which are little to no problem at all. This is the missing ingredient that explains why people who know the calories of certain foods still have problems controlling how much they eat.

Post a Control Value chart on your refrigerator or carry it with your food shopping list. Make a list of the various foods you consume and apply to each food the point system below.

I ABUSE THIS FOOD:

0 = NEVER
1 = RARELY
2 = SOMETIMES
3 = FREQUENTLY
4 = ALWAYS

I ABUSE THIS FOOD:

H = at HOME
W = at the WORKPLACE
S = when STRESSED
B = when BORED
R = at RESTAURANTS
P = around my PERIOD

For example, for you ice cream may earn a rating of 2H, but cookies and chips get a value of 3HWS. The higher the number or the more letters assigned to each food, the greater your control problem. You should strive to avoid any foods scoring a 3 or 4. Here, finally, is an easy, at-a-glance reminder of which foods to eliminate from your kitchen and which to be wary of when outside your home.

VEGETABLES
(1 serving = 1 medium vegetable; one-half cup chopped raw vegetable)

UNLIMITED
all green vegetables	hearts of palm
bean sprouts	mushrooms
eggplant	cauliflower
garlic	summer squash
herbs of all kinds	water chestnuts

LIMITED*
burdock root	rutabagas
jicama	sweet potatoes
kohlrabi	taro root
parsnips	turnips
potatoes	winter squash

USE SPARINGLY, OR AS CONDIMENTS
avocados	onions
beets	peas
carrots	radishes
corn	tomatoes
olives	

*WEIGHT LOSS

WOMEN
1 serving every other day
MEN
1 serving a day

*MAINTENANCE

WOMEN
1 serving a day
MEN
2 servings a day

FRUITS

(1 serving = 1 medium whole fruit; one-half cup chopped fruit; 1 cup berries; one-quarter melon)

FREQUENT

any whole fruit
(except as indicated
below)

any melon (quartered)
grapefruit (halved)

LIMITED

bananas
berries of all kinds

papayas
plantains

USE SPARINGLY, OR AS CONDIMENTS

cherries
coconut
dates

figs
grapes/raisins
watermelon

WEIGHT LOSS	WOMEN
	2 servings a day (1 from "limited")
	MEN
	3 servings a day (1 from "limited")

MAINTENANCE	WOMEN
	3 servings a day (1 from "limited")
	MEN
	2–3 servings a day (1 from "limited")

PROTEIN
(1 serving = 3–5 oz. fish or poultry; 2 oz. solid cheese; 8 oz. yogurt, soft cheese, milk or tofu; 2 oz. sliced meats; 4 oz. lean meat; one-half cup cooked legumes)

FREQUENT

fish	tofu
seafood (all kinds)	nonfat dairy products
poultry (skin removed)	

LIMITED

eggs	reduced-fat dairy products
legumes (beans)	lean beef or veal*
reduced-fat cold cuts	lamb*
reduced-fat hot dogs	reduced-fat pork*

USE SPARINGLY, OR AS CONDIMENTS

prepared meats	whole milk
bacon	high-fat dairy products

WEIGHT LOSS

WOMEN
2 servings a day (1 from "limited")
MEN
3 servings a day (1 from "limited")

MAINTENANCE

WOMEN
2–3 servings a day (1 from "limited")
MEN
2–3 servings a day (1 from "limited")

*Maximum of once a week for men; twice a month for women.

GRAINS

(1 serving = 1 slice bread; one-half cup cooked pasta; one-half cup cooked grains)

LIMITED

protein bread	sugar-free cereals
"light" bread*	brown rice
whole grain or vegetable pastas	other cooked grains

AVOID

white bread	grits
white rice	farina
pastas made with durum, semolina, or other refined flours	any baked goods made with white flour

WEIGHT LOSS	WOMEN 1 serving a day (no pasta or rice) MEN 2 servings a day (pasta or rice once a week)
MAINTENANCE	WOMEN 1–2 servings a day (pasta or rice once a week) MEN 2–3 servings a day (pasta or rice 2–3 times a week)

*40 calories or less per slice

CONDIMENTS

UNLIMITED

horseradish

lemon or lime juice

mustards

picante sauces

salsas

vinegars

LIMITED

nonfat mayonnaise

all-fruit toppings

fruit butters

chutneys

nonfat dressings

vegetable or bean spreads

AVOID

commercial ketchups

commercial dips

commercial salad dressings

mayonnaise

nut butters

THE SUMMER PROBLEM

During the summer months, many of my clients experience what I call the "summer problem." They're eating the right foods, but they're either staying the same weight or seeing the numbers on the scale inch up. They come in upset, perplexed, unable to understand what they're doing wrong. But the answer is really quite simple.

These people are taking advantage of the summer's abundance of fresh produce, keeping ample supplies of grapes, cherries, cut-up melons, and other fruits in their refrigerators. When they actually look at how much and how often they are eating these "healthy, safe" foods, most clients find they are consuming literally pounds of fruit. And although fruit does contain vitamins and other nutrients, it is also high in natural sugars.

The best policy during the high-risk summer months is to abstain entirely from finger fruits, including cut-up fruits such as melon. Instead, enjoy a moderate amount of whole fruits such as peaches, apples, and even halved cantaloupes and other melons. With this relatively simple rule, you can enjoy the bounties of summer without running into the pitfalls of the "summer problem."

Weight Loss: The Basics

Weight loss is a process of persuading your body to give up some of its stored fat. You do this by taking in a little bit less fuel (calories) while putting out a little bit more energy (exercise). When losing weight, it is very important that you eat well and often, so that your body does not go into starvation mode. And it is equally important that you do some sort of exercise so that it is prompted to burn some of that stored fat.

Ultimately, weight loss is a matter of managing calories. Like managing money, it means making wise investments—in foods that give you taste and nutrients without a whopping load of calories.

Those who are most successful at weight loss—the 5 percent who get it off and keep it off—treat their calories like dollars. They don't simply count the calories in food, they look at the quality of the food—how efficiently the body will use the calories the food contains and how many nutrients come with those calories. When faced with the food equivalent of a luxury item—an ice cream sundae, say, or some other fatty dessert—they tend to go for a more economical alternative like fresh fruit, fat-free frozen yogurt, or a sorbet. They don't deny themselves the pleasure of sweet, creamy, or otherwise satisfying foods but they try to choose foods that will give pleasure without unneeded fat, sugar, and calories or losses of control.

While losing weight, you will be eating the same basic foods as after you reach your target weight. But during weight loss you will shift the balance even further away from starchy carbohydrates and grain foods and toward seafood and vegetables. Because the Concorde to weight loss is fish and green vegetables!

If you like ample servings, seafood and vegetables are the way to go. They are low calorie, nutritious, and provide the heart-healthy essential fatty acids your body needs. They are also an excellent way to jump-start your weight loss.

Do Not Skip Meals

This is the most critical rule of the Food Control Eating Plan's weight-loss phase. Skipping meals is the number one predictor of cheating with the wrong foods and slipping back into old out-of-control eating patterns. Even if you slip with a high-calorie snack or meal, don't try to make up for it by skipping your next meal. The meals on the plan are so high in nutrients and low in calories that the occasional slipup will not affect your program.

Skipping meals is both a biological and psychological mistake. Skipping meals sets you up for drops in blood sugar, which leave you hungry and more likely to pick at the very foods you want to avoid. And once you start to substitute picking for eating meals, there is no finish line. A meal is restricted to the plate; but picking turns into a green light for whatever foods you can find in your immediate environment, whether they are trigger foods or not. Whenever my clients report skipping a meal, they also say that they ended up picking at the wrong foods and eating more at the last meal of the day, when the body is least equipped to burn up those extra calories.

Psychologically, once you've skipped a meal it is very easy to fall into negotiation mode. "I didn't eat breakfast," you think, "so maybe it's okay to have this donut." These negotiations almost always involve a food that has a lot more calories and a lot fewer nutrients than the skipped meal, so in the end you always lose out—from both a nutritional and control perspective. So, no matter how busy you are, always eat something at your regular mealtimes—even if it is nothing more than a cup of soup or a high-protein shake.

Eating for Weight Loss

The charts on pages 185–188 list the basic meal and snack options for the weight-loss phase. I have found that most of my clients prefer to have a few simple meals to choose from during the early days of their weight loss. You should feel free to expand on these options with any and all of the recommended foods. Just follow the basic guidelines provided in the pyramids and charts. But remember—after the first week it is not safe to lose more than two pounds per week. If your weight is dropping too fast, increase your intake of starchy vegetables and fruit until your weight loss is in this range.

Breakfast is the first and most important meal of the day, yet it is given short shrift by most people in today's hectic world. You have several breakfast options, all of which can be prepared fast and easily. If you are like many of my clients, you may want to put yourself on automatic pilot in the morning and not deal with making lots of choices. If this is the case, pick one or two options and stick with them. But whatever your choice, make certain you eat *something*.

Those who are carbohydrate sensitive often report that high-carbohydrate breakfasts undermine their control and prompt strong cravings in midmorning. As one of my clients put it, "Whenever I have cereal in the morning I'm ravenous by 10:00 A.M.! I'm better off not eating breakfast at all." If you have a similar problem, you don't need to skip breakfast, you just need to go for a high-protein, low-carbohydrate option.

Lunch can come at almost any time in the afternoon and is generally eaten away from the home, either at restaurants or take-out delicatessens and sandwich shops. Despite the fact that sandwiches are the quintessential lunch foods, I generally don't recommend sandwiches for lunch (or dinner).

Bread products—particularly rolls, bagels, "finger" breads and breads with crunch—are a serious control problem for most people with weight problems. I have found that whenever clients begin reintroducing breads as a regular part of their lunch or dinner menu—even if it is only picking a small piece of crust off a roll in the bread basket—they quickly become habituated to having bread at these meals, and the quantity gradually increases. For this reason, it is better not to associate bread with lunch and dinner. And since most breads are not low calorie, the inclusion of such a high-starch food tends to interfere with weight loss. So limit sandwiches to once a week unless you are losing weight very fast or have absolutely no control problems with bread products. If you need a portable lunch, make sure to use diet, protein, or some other low-calorie bread to make your sandwich.

According to current nutritional wisdom, *dinner* should be the lightest meal of the day because it comes at the end of the body's daily biological cycle when metabolism is at its least efficient. In many European nations, the major meal is in the middle of the day rather than at the end, and—not surprisingly—obesity is less of a problem in these nations.

Unfortunately, in the real world of most Americans' lives, such a pattern is not all that easy to maintain. For most people, dinner comes late and is often the main meal of their busy day. And this tendency is increasing with the rise of two-working-parent and single-parent families, as meals are pushed further and further back because of busy work schedules. So the plan tries to bridge the gap by providing generous dinners that allow dessert and an occasional glass of wine while still being relatively light and low in calories.

Snacking

Although snacks are part of the Food Control Eating Plan, keep in mind that most people gain weight not from calories consumed *at* meals, but from calories consumed *between* meals. If you are a Picker or Prowler, it is important to be aware of when and how much you snack. If you discover that you are becoming hungry in between meals, by all means enjoy the allowed snacks but *schedule* your snacks for specific times in the midmorning, midafternoon, and evening. And *never* include a snack that you've had a history of abusing. If you can't stop at one pudding pop or at a single serving of popcorn, don't try to snack on them.

Many of my clients don't find fruit satisfying and prefer a starchy, crunchy carbohydrate in the afternoon. I recommend that they have a rice cake with a tablespoon or two of no-fat cottage or cream cheese, or, if they have access to a toaster, a fat-free waffle with all-fruit preserves or a slice of toasted light bread. And if, after starting the plan, you dis-

---

THE QUICK AND EASY FOOD CONTROL EATING PLAN

BREAKFAST

- coffee or tea (1 tablespoon low-fat milk allowed)
- 8 oz. nonfat yogurt with 1 tablespoon Grape-Nuts or bran

  OR

  1 fat-free waffle (2 for men) with 2 teaspoons low-calorie syrup, 2 tablespoons all-fruit topping or one-half cup nonfat yogurt

  OR

  single package instant oatmeal or cereal with skim milk and one-half banana or one-half cup berries

  OR

  2 slices toast with 2 wedges nonfat cheese or an egg

  OR

  6 oz. low- or nonfat cottage cheese with piece of fruit

---

cover you're falling into an abusive pattern with one of the recommended foods, switch it out or limit it to restaurants, where servings are controlled. No matter what, remember the lessons of your Eating Print. They won't steer you wrong.

On the other hand, if one of the limited foods is not among your trigger foods, you may want to include it in your eating plan. For example, perhaps you have never had any difficulty losing weight when you have a bagel in the morning. If so, go ahead and have one instead of protein toast or diet bread, so long as it doesn't lead you into eating rolls later in the day.

THE QUICK AND EASY FOOD CONTROL EATING PLAN

LUNCH

- large mixed green salad (dressing on side) or large serving of cooked green vegetable (prepared without oil)
- seltzer, mineral water or diet soda
- individual can of water-packed tuna on bed of greens

  OR

  egg-white omelette

  OR

  5 oz. fish or seafood (prepared without oil)

  OR

  fresh turkey or chicken breast (3 oz. for women, 5 oz. for men) with lettuce and tomato

  OR

  sandwich of 6 slices of "light" cold cuts on low-calorie bread, with mustard or low-fat mayonnaise
- coffee or tea (1 tablespoon of low-fat milk allowed)

Notes: If you find you are not satisfied with these options, add a cup of soup (not cream or bean-based) or a 6 oz. glass of tomato juice.

A small potato or sweet potato can be included in this meal, instead of at dinner.

Special Circumstances: Premenstrual Food Cravings

For many women, the day or two before the menstrual cycle is the time when they are most likely to cheat during weight loss. They experience an increase in appetite, often accompanied by strong cravings for certain foods, particularly chocolate. If you are prone to such cravings, don't panic and don't try to fight or ignore these strong hormonal

---

THE QUICK AND EASY FOOD CONTROL EATING PLAN

DINNER

- mixed green salad
- baked sweet potato or potato
- cooked green vegetable or cup of soup (not cream- or bean-based)
- seltzer, mineral water or diet soda
- grilled chicken breast, skin removed (3 oz. for women, 5 oz. for men)

  OR

  5 oz. any white meat fish (prepared without oil)

  OR

  reduced-fat frankfurters (2 for women, 3 for men) on bed of sauerkraut

  OR

  mixed grilled vegetables with 2 slices nonfat cheese

  OR

  any lunch entrée
- glass of wine or beer (women twice a week, men 3 times a week)
- coffee or tea (1 tablespoon of low-fat milk allowed)

---

messages. Instead, *plan for them!* In the day or so before your period, add a fourth meal to your day, consisting of a large salad with protein (such as tuna) or an extra serving of yogurt. If chocolate cravings are your downfall, add an additional chocolate shake, frozen yogurt, or other allowed chocolate snack. Remember, premenstrual cravings are time limited, and it is far better to work with your biology than to fight it!

Although many of my clients already have had quite a bit of experience choosing low-fat and low-calorie foods, many others feel somewhat at a loss when it comes to picking out specific foods. "Which low-fat cheeses should I

THE QUICK AND EASY FOOD CONTROL EATING PLAN

SNACKS

REQUIRED

fruit (men: 2 servings; women: 1 serving)

plus *one* of the following:

8 oz. nonfat yogurt

4 oz. nonfat frozen yogurt

diet malted or shake

another fruit

fat-free waffle with 1 tablespoon yogurt or all-fruit topping

rice cake or slice of low-calorie toast with nonfat cheese

nonfat popcorn, pre-measured single serving

cup of fat-free soup

OPTIONAL

choose *two:*

diet hot chocolate (25 calories or less)

diet chocolate pop (50 calories or less)

fruit ice pop (70 calories or less)

low-salt instant soup

UNLIMITED

diet beverages

sugar-free gelatin

mineral waters

any "unlimited" vegetable

TROUBLESHOOTING

Healthy weight loss is a steady, gradual process of reshaping and redefining your body. Ideally, you should lose about 2 pounds a week. But everybody (and every *body*) is different, so you may find that your weight loss is not progressing as expected. If you are concerned, try these simple troubleshooting methods.

If you're not losing weight (or losing it too slowly):

- Make sure you're moving. It's not enough just to change your diet. You've got to get moving. Try to exercise at least thirty minutes a day, even if it's only in ten-minute increments.
- Watch out for added salt. Excess sodium causes the body to retain water. Cut back on the salt you add to your meals and switch to fresh lemon, pepper, or other spices.
- Watch out for hidden calories. Make sure your vegetables are steamed or grilled without oil. Order salads with dressing on the side. Try one tablespoon at first and see if it's enough, but don't go beyond two tablespoons per salad. Watch the milk in your coffee and avoid high-calorie nondairy creamers.
- Make sure you get enough liquids. If you're not, your body will respond to the deprivation by retaining fluid. Drink eight to twelve glasses of water a day.
- Don't underestimate your hormones. If you are a woman, some weight gain is normal during the days just before your period. If you seem to be heavier during those days, don't worry about it.
- Be aware of your medications' side effects. Anti-inflammatory drugs, aspirin, hormones, and some antibiotics can prompt water retention and make you think you're not losing weight when you are. If you're concerned, ask your doctor or pharmacist.
- Don't forget about your muscles. If you're exercising regularly, you should be gaining muscle mass even as you lose fat. If the scale seems to be staying put but your clothes are getting looser, then don't worry—you are losing fat even if you don't see a change in the numbers on the scale.

If you are doing everything right and still not losing weight, try making your diet even more white and green by slightly cutting back on starches (flour- and grain-based foods) and fruits.

If you're losing weight too fast:

Make certain you are eating enough. Don't skip meals and make sure you eat all of your allowed snacks. If you're eating all of your allowed meals and snacks, try adding a serving of fruit, root vegetable, or flour-based food every day.

If you're experiencing muscle cramps:

You may be low on potassium. Start eating a banana every day and check with your doctor.

If you're feeling light-headed:

Occasional light-headedness is fairly common in people who are losing weight, particularly when they rise or bend over too abruptly. It is also common in those with low blood pressure. If it persists or happens in other situations, see your doctor.

If you're feeling constipated:

Be sure to drink eight to twelve glasses of water a day and, if it doesn't interfere with your weight loss, try adding a tablespoon of olive oil a day.

If you feel fatigued or headachy during the first few days of weight loss:

If this occurs in midmorning or midafternoon, you may be feeling the effects of a drop in blood sugar. Make sure you have a healthy snack during those times. It's also common for people who once ate large amounts of sweets or starches to experience withdrawal symptoms when they limit these foods. These symptoms can include a day or so of headaches and fatigue. If such symptoms persist, see your doctor.

get?" they ask. "What should I look for in cold cuts?" To make the process easier, my clients and I have put together a listing of some of the better low-calorie, low-fat prepared foods that you can use in creating your menu (see page 295).

The vast majority of my clients have found that losing weight on the Food Control Eating Plan is surprisingly easy. Hopefully you will discover the same thing, particularly as you learn to look beyond the limited foods of your old dietary pattern and start creatively combining the many vegetables, protein sources, and—yes, on occasion—grains that are available to you. For an idea of how much and how well you can eat on my plan, take a look at the sample seven-day diet plan on pages 251–253.

Charting Your Progress

While losing weight, *do not weigh yourself every day.* Get on the scale only once every seven days to track your long-term progress. In general, it is a good idea to weigh yourself in the morning before you have eaten breakfast. After a week, you should begin to see a change in your weight and your shape, particularly if you are exercising.

During the weight-loss phase I also recommend that you maintain a food diary, tracking what and when you eat. Your food diary will enable you to detect any potential problems in your new eating plan and to accurately gauge how much you are eating. If you feel that you are not losing weight fast enough, evaluate your food diary to see if there are any starchy foods that can be cut back.

Maintenance: Living Thin

Once you get to within 5 pounds of your target weight, it is time to switch over to the maintenance phase.

Many people express fears about switching to maintenance before they have reached their target weight. "Keeping it off is the hardest part," they say. "Maybe I should try and lose a few *extra* pounds just in case." These fears are unjustified. If you have been steadily losing weight, your maintenance plan, with its generous portions yet moderate amount of calories, will continue to melt the pounds away. Remember, the Food Control Eating Plan doesn't stop working for you, it helps you move on to another phase in your life of thin.

During maintenance, as during weight loss, white is still light and green is still lean. Your diet will still be based on green vegetables, fish, and poultry, but you can increase your intake of whole grains, an occasional pasta dish, legumes, and alcoholic beverages. In practical terms, this means that you can continue to eat according to the weight-loss plan in general, but allow yourself to have a higher-calorie meal once or twice a week (up to three times a week if you are a man). Treat yourself to a meal at a restaurant or enjoy a dinner at a friend's house. Many of my clients are big fans of olive oil—I encourage them to enjoy one to two tablespoons a day if it is not used in food preparation. When in doubt, look to the maintenance recommendations in the charts.

Besides the charts, there are several things to keep in mind when living thin.

- *You've lost the weight but not the problem.* Your triggers are still your triggers, so continue to use your tapes, Cognitive Switching exercises, and other Food Control Training techniques to help you avoid your triggers and prevent cravings and deprivation.
- *It's not just about calories, it's about control.* Don't

feel that just because a food is low in calories you can automatically reintroduce it into your life. You can't slide back into the old habit of being seduced by low-calorie foods. The essence of Food Control Training is knowing how to evaluate foods based not on calories alone but on cravings and control.

- *Time changes everything.* As we age, metabolic efficiency drops, so we need more nutrients with less calories. For this reason, low-calorie, nutrient-dense foods should become an increasingly important part of your diet as you age. If the pounds start creeping back, increase your intake of fish and green vegetables and cut back on starches.

- *You always need exercise.* Regular exercise is important not only for maintaining your Resting Metabolic Rate, but also for limiting your appetite, increasing your stamina, relieving stress, and giving you all-around good health. When people tell me they eat to relieve stress, I always ask them what other stress outlets they have. Nine times out of ten the answer is none. I always try to steer them in the direction of exercise, because an ever-growing body of evidence indicates that exercise is Nature's Prozac—a powerful (and basically safe) mechanism for improving your mood and outlook on life, as well as your muscle tone. So don't stop exercising just because you're thin.

- *Become a Selective Gourmet.* Success at maintenance is not about food aceticism but about enjoying fine gourmet food with selectivity. As long as you remember that your body has a budget, and you choose your foods accordingly, you can still eat sumptuously.

During maintenance, weigh yourself every other day, preferably in the morning before breakfast. Think of this as a way of keeping track of your investment in thin. It is normal for your weight to vary by a few pounds from day to day, particularly after dining out. Women are also likely to see a few additional pounds in the days immediately preceding the menstrual cycle. But these weight increases should be transient—if your weight is up on Monday, it should be back to normal by Thursday. The time to be concerned is when you show a consistent increase of 3 pounds or more. When this occurs, it's time to evaluate what—and how—you've been eating and go back to the weight-loss plan for a while.

The Food Control Eating Plan is more than just an eating plan for losing weight—it is also an entirely new approach to thinking about and preparing food. To enjoy the diet to its fullest extent, it is therefore important to make some fundamental changes in your approach to *cooking,* changes we will discuss in the next chapter, Cooking for Thin.

COOKING FOR THIN

One cannot live well, love well and sleep well, if one has not dined well.

VIRGINIA WOOLF

I have a confession to make.

Even though I believe that food should always please the palate as much as it protects the waistline . . .

Even though I believe that fresh homemade meals are the most satisfying and healthful . . .

Even though I make a point of living by the dictates of Food Control Training . . .

I rarely cook.

Don't get me wrong. I know *how* to cook! In the days when I was in school and just beginning my practice I often made gourmet dinners for small groups of friends. It was always a pleasure to surprise my guests with rich, delicious, yet low-fat and low-calorie foods. Long before nouvelle cuisine became a byword in the restaurant community, I was steaming vegetables and using broths, wines, and citrus juices to create delicious meals and advising my clients to do the same.

But today my schedule rarely leaves me time to be *near* my kitchen, never mind *in* it! Like many other busy Americans, nowadays I am far more of a Noncook than a Cook.

So, in preparing this chapter, I turned for advice to some people who continue to be active in the world of food preparation. I called upon my clients, who live the Food Control Plan every day, and on chef Susan Knightly, coauthor of *Food for Recovery* (Crown Publishers, 1993) and a true expert at the art of quick, healthy, and delicious cooking. They graciously shared their favorite recipes, cooking techniques, and tricks of the trade and offered invaluable advice. They also suggested several excellent cookbooks that can be used to expand your cooking horizons and recommended favorite recipes from these books to give you a taste of your many options.

Whether you are a Picker or a Prowler, a Noncook or a Cook, the recipes and cooking techniques outlined in this chapter will introduce you to a new world of food where flavor, not fat, is king.

Cooking Made Easy

A meal can be something as grand as beef bourguignonne or as simple as fresh fruit, yogurt, and granola. It can take five hours or five minutes. As one of my clients put it, "Life got a lot easier when I realized that dinner doesn't *have* to be meat and potatoes, breakfast doesn't *have* to be steak and eggs, and lunch doesn't *have* to come precisely at noon. Last night I had a lovely grilled haddock with sautéed green beans. It took about twenty minutes to prepare. It's really too bad my mother didn't know about this. It would have added years to her life outside the kitchen."

To add years to your life outside the kitchen—and make the most of your time in the kitchen—start by following these ten rules of thumb.

1. Keep It Simple. Some of the best meals are made with just a couple of fresh vegetables, some herbs and spices, and a piece of chicken, fish, or even a baked potato.

MORE PEOPLE HAVE GAINED WEIGHT FROM EATING STANDING UP

2. Keep It Quick. Use fast cooking techniques—like steaming, sautéing, or stir-frying—instead of time-intensive methods like roasting or stewing.

3. Spice It Up. Most kitchens contain only a small assortment of herbs and spices—salt, pepper, maybe some garlic powder and oregano—despite the fact that spices from around the world are available at almost any neighborhood supermarket. Expanding your spice rack is the single most important thing you can do to expand your flavor horizons.

4. Be Brave. Once you've got your spices, *use them!* Experiment with combinations to heighten flavor and add a new zest to old foods.

5. Shop Smart. If your vegetables and fish are always fresh, you'll not only find that they are delicious, you will soon discover that your cravings for junk food are fading. If you must use prepared foods, buy the better brands. A good canned vegetable soup, a slice of whole grain bread, and some tuna in spring water is a healthy meal that even the most frazzled person can prepare in minutes. With a good selection of soups, tomato sauces, canned beans, and even frozen dinners (see page 297) in your cupboard and refrigerator you will always have time for a good meal, even when you don't have time to cook.

6. Think Ahead. With a little prior planning in the days and hours when your life is not hectic, you won't be caught off guard during the busy times. Prewash your salad and refrigerate it in a sealed plastic bag. It will stay fresh for a day or two and will make an already fast salad preparation even faster. When preparing beans or grains, double the amount needed and immediately store the extra in ziplock bags in the fridge or freezer for future use. Cooked grains can be used for up to three days and beans for up to four days. And a good broth (see page 255) can last for weeks in the freezer.

7. Invest in a Crock-Pot. Crock-Pots are a great invention. Just put in some vegetables, stock, spices, and poultry (or grains or beans), set the pot on low, leave for the day, and come home to an aromatic soup or stew. You'll find these especially good in the wintertime.

8. Invest in a Steamer. Steaming is one of the quickest and most healthful ways of preparing vegetables and even poultry. A collapsible steamer basket can be used in almost any covered saucepan, or you can purchase a double-layered steamer pot.

9. Invest in a Blender or Food Processor. A sturdy blender or food processor is an invaluable kitchen tool. Simply add ice, yogurt, and fresh fruit, blend, and you've got a thick, frothy shake with none of the calories or cholesterol of ice cream! Or use it to puree vegetables and spices into rich sauces and spreads that can take the place of butter.

10. Ask for Help. What are friends and family for? Enlist aid when you're rinsing or slicing vegetables or preparing a meal. Not only will it make the preparation faster, it will give you a chance to introduce your friends and loved ones to new ways to work in the kitchen.

All of these tricks can make cooking healthy meals fast and simple. But *eating* those meals should never be fast. Sit down and enjoy your meals, instead of wolfing them down on the run.

Getting Away from Fat

Americans love to cook with fat. From chicken-fried steak to french-fried potatoes to fried chicken to deep-fried zucchini sticks, if it can be immersed in hot oil, we find a way to do it. But there is an entire world of cooking that does not revolve around oil and fat. In gourmet and not-so-gourmet kitchens around the world, cooks of every description regularly make extraordinary meals that require little or no oil or fat. Indeed, these techniques are rapidly taking over the restaurant world. But you don't have to become a professional chef or pay a hundred dollars for a meal at a trendy French restaurant to enjoy the taste and health benefits of these cooking techniques. You just need to broaden your horizons a bit.

The popularity of oils, butter, and lard—and their artificial equivalents like margarine—is rooted in two things, flavor and moisture. Butter and cooking oils not only impart their own particular flavor to food, they can also be heated to a level that seals moisture into the delicate tissues of meats, vegetables, and even some fruits. Unfortunately, few cooks realize that they can enjoy these benefits with only a tiny amount of oil. If they did, deep-fat fryers would have gone the way of the eight-track tape years ago.

The one cooking technique that does require at least a little oil is sautéing, or stir-frying. (Technically, stir-frying refers to cooking in a wok, but since you can stir-fry food in any deep skillet, I will use the terms interchangeably.) Sautéed or stir-fried foods are cooked fast over high heat and kept in constant motion. This technique preserves foods' flavor, crispness, and nutrients and is a particularly fast and easy way to prepare vegetables.

The single drawback of stir-frying and sautéing is the tendency of most cooks to overoil the pan. Sautéed and stir-fried foods should never swim in oil. Use just enough oil to lubricate the pan. A thin layer of oil, along with your constant stirring and tossing, is more than enough to prevent the food from sticking to the pan during the few minutes it takes to cook. To keep yourself from falling into the excess oil trap when stir-frying or sautéing, try these simple tricks:

- *Measure!* Instead of pouring oil directly into the pan, measure it out by the teaspoon or tablespoon.
- *Spray!* Spraying oil onto a pan guarantees a light, even coating. You can use one of the dozens of commercial cooking sprays or make your own by pouring your favorite cooking oil into an inexpensive plastic spray bottle. One warning, though—sprays can be deceptive. Only the thinnest coating of oil is needed, so don't be heavy-handed. If you aren't careful, you can add several tablespoons of oil to your "low-fat" dish.
- *Wipe!* The ultimate way to be certain you haven't overoiled your pan is to wipe up the excess. Warm the pan a bit and wipe away the excess that accumulates as the heated oil becomes more liquid. You'll still have more than enough to prevent sticking.

In addition to stir-frying, there are several "dry" cooking techniques that work very well for fish, poultry, and vegetables of all kinds. Grilling (cooking over high heat) and broiling (cooking under high heat) both allow extra fat to drain away from foods while giving them the crispy texture we normally associate with frying. Both methods work particularly well with marinated meats and vegetables. Baking or roasting surrounds food with a more even heat and allows subtle flavors to blend and develop slowly, particularly when the food is kept covered (usually with aluminum foil) during the early stage of cooking.

Cooking with Liquids

Any food that can be cooked in oil can be prepared in other nonfat liquids. From plain water to fine wines, liquids can be used to braise, poach, blanch, steam, and even stir-fry almost any food.

Broths (or stocks) are an excellent way of adding flavor, nutrients, and moisture to food without adding fat. They can be the foundation for tasty soups and sauces, and can be used to cook any grain or bean. (A warning, though—never use salt in broths used for cooking dried beans. Your beans will remain hard forever.)

Although commercially prepared broths are available, these canned products often have a high salt content. Read labels carefully and when in doubt, go for one of the better name brands, such as Health Valley, Hains, or Eden Farm. Some of the larger food companies (such as Campbell's and Progresso) are now offering reduced-salt/reduced-fat soups and broths as well, so keep your eye out for these healthful options.

Keep in mind, though, that if you can boil water you can make your own broth, using whatever you have in the house. Making vegetable broth is as easy as putting a few vegetables into a pot of water and turning on the flame. (Avoid using cabbage, broccoli, and other cruciferous greens. Their flavor is so strong that it can overpower the broth.) Add some chicken or beef bones and voilà, you've got chicken or beef broth! (When making meat or poultry

---

ONE CHIP, BUT HOW MANY CHIPS YOU EAT ✧ "NO FAT" DOESN'T MEAN

broths, be sure to let the broth cool so you can skim off any congealed fat.) Homemade broths can be frozen or just re-frigerated and can last for weeks.

Wines and spirits have a long and distinguished history in cooking. Red and white wines, sherries, vermouth, and certain hard liquors like vodka and brandy lend a new di-mension to many dishes. And since much of the alcohol evaporates during cooking, these spirits add their distinc-tive flavors without adding calories. As a result, alcoholic beverages are among the most popular liquids used in nou-velle cuisine. When working with wines and other liquors, follow these basic rules.

- Use a wine good enough to drink on its own. If it doesn't taste good in the wineglass, it won't taste good in your meal.
- Add wine toward the end of cooking, when sauces or stir-frys are just about done. This will ensure that the flavor comes through.
- Be subtle. Spirits can overwhelm other flavors if you add too much. Add wine or other liquors in small in-crements and check for taste before adding more. Be especially conservative with sherries, whiskey, and brandies. They have very strong, distinctive tastes, and a little will go a long way.
- In marinades, use wines and other light spirits (such as vodka and vermouth).
- For poached dishes, try adding dry white wine or ver-mouth.

One note of caution—for those in recovery from alcohol or drug addiction, even a hint of alcohol may reactivate old cravings. If you are concerned about these issues, or know that one or more of your guests are in recovery, stick to one of our other liquid cooking tools.

Vinegar may be the most underrated of all condiments. If your use of vinegar is limited to the salad bowl, then you've been missing out on one of the best cooking tools around. In addition to its unique zing, vinegar has a particular talent for absorbing the flavors of herbs, spices, vegetables, and fruits. These infused or herbed vinegars add real sizzle to chicken, fish fillets, or even the blandest vegetables. Herbed vinegars can be used in place of oil when stir-frying or sautéing, or they can be added to a dish as it is cooking to add a subtle sparkle of aroma and flavor. They make terrific marinades, and of course they're perfect for salad dressings.

Prepared herbed vinegars are now widely available, so it's easy to stock your kitchen with a selection. Or you can make your own, using quality vinegar and your own fresh herbs. If you're unsure about which foods will work best with infused vinegars, follow these guidelines at first and then branch out as your imagination (and taste buds!) expand:

- Use chive or tarragon vinegars with chicken, fish, green beans, and white beans.
- Use basil or garlic vinegars with eggplant, tomatoes, zucchini, greens, and chicken.
- Use dill vinegar with beets, whole greens, yellow squash, and fish.
- Use rosemary or allspice vinegars with root vegetables, chicken, and tuna.
- Use ginger vinegar with broccoli, curry dishes, and stir-frys.

YOU CAN'T HAVE EVERYTHING YOU WANT, YOU CAN STILL HAVE

Preparing Vegetables

Vegetables are the mainstay of the Food Control Eating Plan, and with good reason. They are an invaluable source of vitamins, minerals (including calcium), fiber, and even protein, all at a remarkably low caloric cost. Depending on how they are prepared, vegetables can satisfy your taste for crunch or for creaminess as well as satisfying your need to enjoy generous servings.

Most green vegetables work equally well when served hot or cold, and almost any leafy vegetable—including raw cabbage—can be used as the base for salads, the simplest and yet most versatile way of serving fresh vegetables.

For many people (and some restaurants) a salad is little more than a few pieces of iceberg lettuce and some sliced tomato. But the true diversity of salads knows no limit. Almost any vegetable that is served hot—from artichokes to zucchini—will work in a salad. Add a few ounces of protein—in the form of tuna, shrimp, grilled chicken, or even tofu—and you have a nutritionally complete, thoroughly delicious meal.

Salads are also the place to add whole grains, pastas, and legumes to your menu without running into the serving-size dilemma that makes these foods such a control problem. A half cup of cooked pasta, beans, or barley looks considerably more generous when it is mixed into a heaping platter of greens than when it is huddled off to the side of a dinner plate.

The sole drawback of salads is in the dressing. Pre-dressed salads often swim in oil-based dressings that can add hundreds of calories to these normally low-calorie meals. Even a relatively low-calorie, low-fat dressing, such as those listed on page 300, can become a problem if you pour too much onto your greens.

Most salads are simply delicious when dressed with nothing more fancy than some lemon juice or balsamic vinegar. When using these and other low-fat salad dressings, there are ways to get around the problem of overuse.

- First and foremost, never order (or serve) a salad predressed. Have the dressing on the side so you (and your guests) can know exactly how much dressing you are adding.
- You can also assure a modest, even distribution of salad dressing by using a spray bottle rather than pouring. Richard Simmons pioneered this concept with his Salad Sprays, but you can make your own with your favorite dressing and an inexpensive spray bottle. (One warning, though—the spray option won't work with chunkier dressings!)

Blanching is a great technique for preparing vegetables you want to serve crisp and cold as part of a salad or as crudités. It cooks vegetables just enough to heighten their color and soften the tough outer layer but keeps them crisp enough to still give that satisfying crunch. Simply plunge the sliced vegetables briefly into boiling water, drain immediately, and then plunge them into cold water to stop the cooking process. The vegetables will be bright, crisp, and just tender enough. Blanching works particularly well with broccoli, cauliflower, carrots, zucchini, green beans, and asparagus.

For hot vegetables, *steaming* may be the easiest (and most popular) preparation technique. With a covered saucepan, a steam basket, some vegetables, and some water or broth, you can prepare delicious vegetables with even more speed than a microwave. Simply place the vegetable-filled steam basket in a pot containing an inch or so of boiling water, cover, and wait. Within minutes (and I do mean minutes! Be careful not to overcook.) you'll have an ample serving of hot fresh vegetables, perfect for serving over brown rice, a baked potato, or alongside some broiled fish or chicken. To heighten the flavor of your steamed vegetables, add some garlic, onions, or other herbs and spices to the mix.

Stir-frying requires a little more work than steaming but is worth the effort. Stir-fried vegetables come out bright, crisp, and delicious—satisfying that need for something crunchy and hot. When stir-frying, make sure you begin with a very hot, lightly oiled wok or large frying pan. (Note: The oil should *not* smoke in the pan.) If using garlic or onions, briefly sauté them first until the onions are translucent. Then add the tougher vegetables—such as cabbage, broccoli, cauliflower, or carrots—so they can cook thoroughly. Add softer vegetables—such as zucchini, eggplant, mushrooms, or yellow squash—just as the colors of the first vegetables are brightening.

Stir-frying is fast, so remember to keep the vegetables in constant motion to prevent sticking. If they start to stick, do not add oil. Add a splash of broth, wine, or vinegar instead—it will lubricate the pan, and as it evaporates, it will add flavor and moisture to your cooking vegetables.

Grilling—either from above (technically broiling) or below—gives marinated vegetables a wonderful crispy exterior and tender flavorful interior. Grilled vegetables make excellent hors d'oeuvres, appetizers, or main dishes and are equally delicious hot or cold.

The recipes beginning on page 268 will work with almost any mix of vegetables, so enjoy experimenting.

Preparing Seafood and Poultry

Seafood and poultry (particularly chicken and turkey) are important sources of protein in the Food Control Eating Plan. They can be grilled, stir-fried, and even steamed just as easily as vegetables, although they require a little more time to be thoroughly cooked. In addition to these methods, you may also want to try two other simple cooking techniques, poaching and braising.

Poaching is an excellent alternative to frying for eggs, chicken, and some types of fish. (Beef is not a candidate for poaching, however.) Food is simmered in a shallow layer (enough to almost cover its surface) of water or other liquid until thoroughly cooked. Although special poaching racks exist (and can be particularly useful when poaching eggs), they are not a necessity. To add flavor, you can often poach foods on a layer of diced onions and herbs and use the flavorful liquid as a sauce. Foods poached in wine or broth can have just as much flavor as foods fried in butter, and they are considerably more kind to your arteries!

Braising is one of the most flavorful fat-free cooking methods. Chicken or tougher cuts of meat can be braised by cooking with a small amount of liquid in a tightly covered pan over very low heat. Braising also works well with vegetables—try it with celery in vegetable broth for a real taste surprise.

Dressing It Up Without Adding Fat

The proper use of herbs and spices can turn a simple meal of chicken and vegetables into something spectacular. If your seasonings have been limited to salt, pepper, and a handful of dried herbs, expand your horizons. Most supermarkets now carry fresh herbs (such as dill, cilantro, basil, and parsley) in addition to the dried variety, and these fragrant greens complement a wide range of foods.

In addition to fresh options, you also may want to consider some of the better seasoning blends. These prepared spices are a quick way to add flavor to seafood, vegetables, and poultry. For just the right combination of spices and dried herbs without excess sugar or monosodium glutamate (MSG), try chef Paul Prudhomme's Magic Seasoning Blends—Seafood Magic, Poultry Magic, and Vegetable Magic—anything from Mrs. Dash, or Bookbinder's Restaurant Style Crab & Shrimp Seasoning.

Although spices can add flavor and piquancy to the plainest of foods, they cannot provide the satisfying "mouth feel" associated with the textures of creamy sauces and gravies. The prospect of giving up such pleasures caused some of my clients dismay—until they learned of the many low-fat nontrigger foods that can satisfy the palate as well as creamy sauces once did.

Good substitute foods give you the flavors and textures you enjoy without using buckets of cream, pounds of cheese, or bags of sugar. Many of the larger food companies have developed new low-fat versions of classically high-fat foods—including cheese—that are just as tasty and satisfying as the old versions. There are also scores of soups, salad dressings, mayonnaises, and various other condiments that have dramatically reduced fat levels. These products can be used to give your meals the textures you crave without adding the fat you want to avoid.

Low-fat dairy products like cottage cheese and plain yogurt work well in the place of higher-fat products such as whole milk ricotta cheese and sour cream. Ground turkey or chicken works well in burgers, "meat" loaf, or just about any dish that requires ground beef. But be wary—most prepackaged turkey or chicken "burgers" include skin, dark meat, and various other high-fat, high-calorie portions of the bird. If you want to use ground poultry, buy the meat and ask the butcher to grind it for you.

If you are feeling adventurous, you can also go entirely outside of the traditional meat and dairy groups and look to some of the vegetable kingdom's "great pretenders."

Perhaps the greatest of these is *tofu,* a cheeselike curd made from soybeans. Tofu's light delicate flavor and adaptable texture (from silky soft to firm and chewy) make it the perfect substitute for everything from ground beef to whipping cream. And unlike beef *or* cream, tofu provides calcium and protein without a whopping load of saturated fat and cholesterol.

Tofu comes in two forms: a firm curd that can be scrambled like eggs or marinated and roasted like meat, and a silky soft variety that works well when pureed and used in place of cream. Both varieties can be used as cheese substitutes in quiches, cheesecakes, lasagna, and more.

Most major supermarkets now carry tofu, either loose or packaged, so you can easily purchase and experiment with this remarkable food. One pound of tofu equals about two cups. It should be fresh and snowy white, not pink or bubbly. Tofu can be stored—covered in water—in the refrigerator for several days as long as you change the water each day; it freezes remarkably well. Consider using tofu in place of eggs, chicken, or any meat in stir-frys. Try marinating firm slices of tofu in your favorite herb vinegar before adding it to stir-frys. Experiment with pureed tofu as a base for dips and sauces, mixing it with flavored vinegar, herbs, and chopped vegetables.

Like tofu, root vegetables and beans of any kind can be pureed and served up as rich sauces to accompany chicken, fish, beef, or cooked vegetables and grains. Unlike flour, cream, or other thickening agents, these "pretenders" actually raise the nutritional content of your meal—adding fiber, vitamins, minerals, and (in the case of beans) all-important protein.

Whipped sweet potatoes with nutmeg and cinnamon can serve as an elegant accompaniment to meat and chicken dishes. Pureed potatoes can be used to thicken soups or sauces of any kind. Pureed black beans make an excellent sauce for chicken, while pureed white beans make delicious low-fat "cream" sauces that can be used with almost any poultry, meat, whole grain, or fish.

Guilt-Free Desserts

I've heard it dozens of times. A client, after reviewing her Eating Print and identifying her trigger foods, looks at me in dismay and says, "So if I'm going to stay thin, I'll never be able to eat dessert again, right?"

Wrong. Living thin does not mean living without the pleasure of an occasional sweet, creamy, or crunchy dessert item. Once you've reached your target weight and have established the parameters of your boxes you can even occasionally have one of your old favorites. But for the most part, you can satisfy your desire for dessert without feeling guilt-ridden simply by being creative.

Fruits are nature's dessert—and with some imagination, time, and a blender you can turn your daily allowance of fruit into creamy frozen desserts, mouthwatering pies, and fat-free shakes that will satisfy even the most avid ice cream addicts. You can also add fruit to some of the excellent fat-free frozen desserts for a healthy alternative to ice cream sundaes.

The major food companies have shown particular ingenuity in coming up with low-calorie versions of cakes, cookies, ice creams, frozen pops, and just about any other dessert you can imagine. Most of these products do indeed taste good and they are great alternatives to high-fat, high-calorie options when you are entertaining. But don't fall into the trap of keeping these nonfat foods in your home, particularly if you have a history of abusing them. You will get just as fat on the low-fat version as you did on the high-fat one—it will just take a little longer. When in doubt, use fruit to satisfy your dessert needs.

The techniques presented in this chapter (and the recipes beginning on page 255) are only the beginning of what you can do with the almost unlimited selection of healthy foods that are available at your local supermarket. Once you begin enjoying the taste benefits of this kind of cooking, you'll find it hard to go back.

Many of my clients were amazed at how easy it was to make the switch, and even more amazed at how well their families and dinner guests responded to it. Children who refused to have anything to do with vegetables were asking for seconds of roasted zucchini and peppers. Husbands who would never willingly eat beans were singing the praises of swordfish in white bean sauce. Guests who used to empty bowls of chips were now emptying platters of veggie kabobs and hounding them for recipes. In the words of one particularly surprised (but pleased) Food Control Training hostess, "As long as it tastes good, no one cares if it's made from tofu or lard, sweet potatoes or cornstarch. Everyone keeps asking me how I lost so much weight on all these delicious foods. All I can tell them is, try it, it will work for you too."

EATING OUT AND ON THE RUN

The customer is always right.
AMERICAN ADAGE

Up until a couple of decades ago, eating at home was the norm and eating out was a rare treat. Nowadays, almost the exact reverse is true. Most people eat at least one meal outside the home each day, and some people routinely eat all three of their major meals while out or on the run.

Eating out doesn't have to mean eating badly. Most restaurants—from the most expensive five-star establishment to the most humble diner—have caught on to the trend toward healthy low-fat foods and have made adjustments accordingly. Choosing these dishes, and making a few simple requests, can make eating out a healthy as well as convenient experience.

General Guidelines

The greatest danger of eating in restaurants isn't the entrée, it's the breads, chips, and other foods that most restaurants ply customers with *before* the entrée is even ordered. How many times have you gone out to dinner and found yourself saying, "I'm not even hungry anymore," when the entrée arrived, all because you had stuffed yourself on bread or some other appetizer? And how often did you go ahead and eat the entrée anyway?

You can save yourself a lot of grief and temptation by doing one of two things. First, never go to a restaurant hungry. The same golden rule that applies to dinner or cocktail parties is most applicable when dining at any commercial establishment. If you are starving when you arrive, you know what will happen. The first thing brought to the table is the bread basket and you will dive right in. There is a natural inclination to pick. If ever there is a place where finger control is important, it is at a restaurant.

Second, simply tell your server that you would prefer not to have a bread basket on the table. If your dinner companions want bread, turn your bread plate over, ask them to keep the bread basket on the other side of the table, or ask the waiter to remove the basket after everyone has taken what they want. You may find, as I have, that others share your susceptibility to the temptations of the bread basket and are only too happy to have it gone.

The same goes for the little cookies or mints that some restaurants serve with coffee or dessert. Ask the waiter about it in advance. You needn't feel embarrassed or timid about such requests. More and more people are making these requests every day. Invariably, a good waiter always appreciates anything specific you can tell him about what you need to keep you pleased and satisfied.

When it comes to ordering beverages, mineral water is better than club soda from a nutritional perspective—have it with lemon or lime.

Don't let the menus tempt you. Some people find that reading the menu sabotages them and makes them crave. You can just ignore the menu and ask the waiter for a simply prepared grilled chicken breast. Or ask the waiter for his recommendation on the best fish entrée in the house. Or just keep your reading to the chicken and fish sections of the menu. Dining out should be fun and a rewarding experience. Don't deny yourself this joy because you are afraid to read the dessert section on a menu.

Predressed salads are a big source of hidden calories, since most restaurants tend to drown their healthy green salads in less-than-healthy oil-based dressings. To control the amount of dressing, request your salad with dressing on the side and choose a vinaigrette dressing.

When ordering your entrée, steer clear of foods that are prepared with heavy sauces or gravies. Instead look for dishes that have been prepared without butter, cream, and other fatty condiments. For example, order foods that have been:

- baked (*without* rich sauces or gravies)
- grilled (without oil)
- broiled (without oil)
- poached
- roasted
- steamed

Always ask if you can have your dish prepared without the sauce—or with wine or broth rather than butter. If ordering a steak or other cut of beef, make a point of requesting that all excess fat be trimmed before cooking. Most good restaurants are very willing to accommodate such requests.

If you aren't sure about a restaurant's policies concerning special requests, call in advance. Find out if entrées can be modified. Ask if chicken and other meats have their fat removed before cooking. If the restaurant isn't willing to give you this kind of information or is unwilling to make modifications in its menu for individual customers, you may want to think about dining somewhere else.

When choosing desserts, keep moderation in mind. It is perfectly fine during the Maintenance phase to have an occasional piece of cake or other sweet dessert if it is not one of your critical trigger foods. But keep in mind that most restaurants now offer fruit, sorbet, sherbet, or other fruit-based desserts that can satisfy your sweet tooth with far less fat and calories. When in doubt, choose the fresh fruit options.

Below, I've provided some specific advice on what to do in some of the most popular ethnic restaurants.

Eating Italian

With the new Mediterranean Diet garnering praise from health researchers, it makes more sense than ever before to check out your local *ristorante italiano.* You still have to be careful when ordering, considering Italian chefs' predilection for liberal quantities of olive oil. (Keep in mind that although olive oil is one of the better cooking oils, it is still a fat, and very high in calories. As I tell my clients, "It may be good for you, but it's not good for your weight.") But even so, there are many delicious, low-fat, and filling Italian foods, all of which you can enjoy while dining out.

The "bread basket rule" is particularly important in Italian restaurants. Beware of garlic bread—it is a major villain when it comes to the Aroma Problem. The Aroma Problem, i.e., the fact that smells can be compelling appetite triggers, is always troubling when eating out, but especially so at Italian restaurants and—even worse—pizzerias. Perhaps you have taken your children to a pizzeria with the best intentions, but the aromas strike first, then the vision of the pizza as it comes fresh out of the oven, acting like a one-two punch to your resolve. But you know what to do now.

You remind yourself what you're smelling—it's the smell of fat.

When ordering entrées, most people don't realize that with a little guidance, you can get the chef to cook nouvelle Italian, using broth or wine instead of oil. If you are having a dish that is broiled, ask that the chef use wine or lemon rather than oil when preparing your meal. Or see if it can be grilled with little or no oil at all.

While pasta is often touted as a good diet food, it is anything but low calorie when laden with sauce and cheese. Avoid white sauces (which are packed with cream and cheese) and pesto sauces (which are usually very oily) and choose instead marinara, pomidoro, or other tomato-based sauces. When in doubt, decline the addition of cheeses such as grated Parmesan.

And to truly stay in control, request an appetizer or half-sized portion, or split a meal with a friend.

Choosing Chinese

Chinese foods are a bit of a paradox from the Food Control Training perspective. On the one hand, many Chinese dishes are wonderful light collections of flavorful vegetables and whole grains. On the other hand, many are deep-fried, laden with sugar, or covered with cornstarch-thickened sauces. Differentiating between these types of dishes is important.

First and foremost, ask what is in any given dish. Are the sauces made with cornstarch? Are the noodles prepared with oil or without? Is the rice whole brown rice or steamed white rice? (If the latter, don't order it.) Are the vegetables fried or steamed? Can they be prepared without fat? After numerous accounts in the media about how high in fat some Chinese dishes can be, Chinese restaurants are starting to be more creative with low-cal, low-fat cooking. Many will now sauté your foods in wine, scallions, and ginger, which many feel gives a richer taste to vegetables than mere steaming. It's simply a matter of making your needs known. All restaurant managers want return customers; if they know how to make foods for you that are delicious and healthful, they know you'll be back.

Many good Chinese restaurants pride themselves on serving healthy dishes, so you should be able to find several good, low-fat options on the menu. However, the crispy noodles and duck sauce that are usually placed on the table are NOT a good low-fat option. They are, in fact, packed with fat, sugar, and cornstarch, and you should ask to have them removed.

Eating Mexican

Mexican restaurants were all the rage in the 1980s and are still quite popular in most cities. The traditional rice and bean dishes of Mexico are excellent sources of complete protein and fiber, but the rice and beans served in most Mexican restaurants are not. The beans are usually prepared with far too much fat, and the rice has been so highly refined that its nutrients are nonexistent. And Mexican restaurants often drown their dishes in cheese.

That doesn't mean you can't enjoy an occasional Mexican meal, however. Vegetable, beef, and chicken fajitas can usually be prepared with a minimum of fat on request. Enchiladas and burritos can be served with tomato-based salsa or *pico de gallo* (a mix of tomatoes, onions, and hot peppers) and without additional cheese. Simply be sure to ask your server to specify that you don't want the refried beans or cheese. (And, of course, steer clear of those chips!)

YES, VIRGINIA, THERE IS LOW-CAL MEXICAN

The Center for Science in the Public Interest (CSPI) surveyed the cuisine at a host of Mexican eateries and was hard-pressed to find anyplace that didn't go overboard on fat and sodium—till they came to the Pacific Northwest. In the Seattle and Portland areas they discovered Macheezmo Mouse, a chain that actually turns out low-fat Mexican dishes, with the help of brown rice, no-fat black beans, lower-fat cheese, whole wheat tortillas, marinated veggies, sour cream blended with nonfat yogurt, and a broad selection of salads with low-fat dressing. These are the kinds of suggestions you can make to the manager of your own favorite Mexican restaurant. Or write to Macheezmo and get them to open a branch near you.

Eating on the Plane

Airline foods aren't known for being particularly tasty or particularly healthful. In fact, recent surveys of the nutritional content of regular airline meals found that up to 50 percent of their calories were from fat—hardly a healthy eating experience.

Fortunately, you can improve your in-flight dining experience by making a phone call in advance. Airlines are quite accommodating to passengers with specific dietary restrictions or desires, and will arrange to have a special meal waiting for you on the plane as long as you let them know about it a few days ahead of time. The specific deadlines differ from airline to airline, so check when you book your ticket.

If you ask, most airlines will provide you with sample menus of their various special meals. In general, the low-cholesterol meals are a good bet, as are the diabetic and kosher meals. Be careful when ordering vegetarian meals,

---

since they often rely on pasta. Try to get a sample menu before you make your decision.

Of course, the simplest alternative is to bring your own food. A perfect choice would be fruit, low-fat cheese, a diet bread sandwich, or perhaps a cup of yogurt with Grape-Nuts or granola. And need I mention this? Watch out for the peanuts and pretzels. Just have some soda (and ask for the whole can if they offer only a cupful) or a can of tomato juice—this should help quell any hunger pangs till you land.

Eating on the Road

Once upon a time, renting a room in a hotel meant just that, renting a *room*. Today, many hotel rooms come equipped with their own minirestaurants in the form of in-room refrigerators and wet bars. Unfortunately, they are usually stocked with precisely the types of foods you want to avoid. And since travel has become a high-stress activity, you are usually very vulnerable, especially when you first arrive in your room.

You can protect yourself from such sources of temptation in several ways. When checking in, request a room without a fridge or wet bar. If that isn't possible, and the in-room refrigerator has a separate lock, don't accept the key. Or, failing that, ask the concierge to have everything but the diet sodas and mineral waters removed from the refrigerator before you take the room. Also be sure to ask whether housekeeping leaves mints or chocolates on the pillows. If so, ask that they not do so in your room.

Such requests are much easier to accommodate if you give the hotel some advance notice, so if you know where you will be staying, make these arrangements at the time you book the room.

Navigating the Fast-Food Wilderness

The most popular places for out-of-the-home eating are not hotels, airplanes, or even restaurants. They are fast-food outlets. From Arby's to Hardee's, from McDonald's to Burger King, millions upon millions of Americans get their meals daily from these fast-food giants.

Amazing as it may seem, despite the fact that many of their foods are high in fat, sugar, and calories, it *is* possible to eat a relatively healthy meal at a fast-food outlet. Most of the major chains have responded to the call for more healthy foods by adding salad bars, soups, and a variety of reduced-fat sandwiches to their menus. They still carry the old favorites, of course, but now you have a choice.

My personal favorite is Arby's Light Roast Chicken Deluxe sandwich. You can eliminate the roll if you want and substitute a salad (or try their delicious Roast Chicken Salad). It is tasty, nutritious, and inexpensive. Burger King has a grilled chicken breast and McDonald's a salad with chunks of chicken that are also quite good.

If french fries or burgers have always haunted you in the past, decide before you go in what you are ordering, so you won't be tempted while waiting on line. Give the new salad bars and light menus a try. Just keep the following caveats in mind:

- Most condiments (like bacon bits, croutons, and grated cheeses) are not low calorie or low fat. Steer clear of them.
- Creamy salad dressings are also a big must to avoid. Stick to the vinaigrettes and use them sparingly.

Some people find it easy just to avoid these places entirely. But that may not be a workable option for you if you have children. If all else fails, remember that you can wait in the car while your kids go in to order their lunches. Or if the children are very young, then be aware of the major problem that families have when going out for fast food: Mom or Dad finishing up the kids' leftovers. If you can keep control over that and choose something healthy and low-fat for your own lunch, then the fast-food dining experience should be no more problematic than eating anywhere else.

In the table below, I have listed some of the better food

FAST-FOOD BEST BETS

Name of Chain/Menu Item	Calories	% of Calories from Fat
Arby's (800-487-ARBY)		
Grilled Chicken Barbecue Sandwich	386	30
Side Salad w/ Light Italian Dressing	48	26
Light Roast Beef Deluxe Sandwich	294	30
Light Roast Turkey Deluxe Sandwich	260	21
Light Roast Chicken Deluxe Sandwich	276	23
Old-Fashioned Chicken Noodle Soup	99	16
Burger King (800-937-1800)		
BK Broiler Chicken Sandwich	280	32
Chef Salad w/ Light Italian Dressing	303	3
Chunky Chicken Salad w/ Light Italian Dressing	288	15
Garden Salad w/ Light Italian Dressing	253	21

Name of Chain/Menu Item	Calories	% of Calories from Fat
Hardee's (800-346-2243)		
Turkey Sub	390	16
Roast Beef Sub	370	12
Ham Sub	370	17
Combo Sub	380	14
Grilled Chicken Breast Sandwich	310	26
McDonald's (708-575-3663)		
Chunky Chicken Salad w/ 1 T Lite Vinaigrette Dressing	162	25
Fat-Free Apple Bran Muffin	180	0
Vanilla Lowfat Frozen Yogurt Cone	105	8
Subway (Nutritional Division, 325 Bic Drive, Milford, CT 06460)		
Six Inch Veggies & Cheese Sub (without dressing or mayo)	258	22
Six Inch Roast Turkey Breast Sub (without dressing or mayo)	312	22

choices from the major fast-food chains. These companies will gladly send you a complete nutritional breakdown of their menus to help guide your food choices.

Whenever you eat outside the home, your food choices should be governed by the same rules that dictate your choices in the supermarket and in your own kitchen. Stay away from your trigger foods and choose foods that are high in nutrients but low in calories. That means choosing the freshest, least adulterated food available—whether it's a green salad at Arby's or steamed vegetables in garlic sauce at your favorite Chinese restaurant. Whatever you choose, you will soon discover that healthy eating can be just as enjoyable and delicious as eating fat-, calorie-, and salt-laden food.

A FINAL TIP . . .

For more information on healthy choices when eating out, check out *The Living Heart Guide to Eating Out* by world-renowned heart surgeon Dr. Michael E. DeBakey, Dr. Antonio Gotto, Jr., and nutrition expert Lynne W. Scott. This pocket-sized book contains terrific tips on how to eat healthy when dining at everything from Cajun to Vietnamese restaurants. It's available at most bookstores or call (713) 798-4150.

LIVING IN A HOUSE OF FOOD

*A house full of people is a house full of
different points of view.*
MAORI PROVERB

Part of Food Control Training is learning to live—and
maintain control—in a world of food, a world with other
people, a world in which other people's wishes and desires
won't always agree with yours. But you can educate those
around you and take steps to make your home environment,
if not trigger-free, then at least fairly safe.

Sometimes clients will say that they can't keep their trigger foods out of the house because it's not fair to their family. Or they try to justify keeping some of their triggers
around because "food is everywhere—I have to learn to
live with it." These rationales are very considerate, rational,
even logical. But they're still wrong.

It is one thing to know your triggers are out there in the
world and quite another to have them right under your nose.
There's nothing you can do about the high-fat or high-calorie foods that are in the local pizzeria or fast-food places,
but you don't have to live with them in your own house. If
you could live with them, you wouldn't have a weight problem. So don't try to tempt yourself. Recovering alcohol or
drug addicts don't keep Scotch or cocaine around just to
test their resolve. Why should you?

As far as depriving the other members of your household goes, take a moment to assess who is *really* applying the pressure. Is your spouse, child, or roommate the one who can't live without those Ring-Dings in the house or is it you? More often than not, my clients end up discovering that *they,* not other members of their households, are the ones who are bringing the foods in.

Even if some members of your household grouse about not having twenty-four-hour access to potato chips, keep your perspective. If you were recovering from alcoholism, no true friend or loved one would insist on keeping a fully stocked bar in the house against your wishes. If you were an insulin-dependent diabetic they would not ply you with candy bars. If you were allergic to shellfish they would not serve you crab cakes. Human beings regularly make concessions to protect the health and well-being of those they care about.

If you have children, this is one of the most powerful lessons you can ever teach them about empathy and the welfare of another human being. After all, one of the central missions of a family is to impart a sense of caring and love to each of its members. When you explain to your children that certain foods are a problem for you, their parent, it teaches them an awareness that mothers and fathers also have growth issues that they are working on. If you take the food out of the house in an arbitrary and authoritarian way, you are sure to be greeted with squawks, complaints, and resentment. But there is no squawking when you make the child a participant in a caring act for a family member.

Keeping your trigger foods out of your home environment is not an unreasonable condition as long as you make it clear to household members *why* you need to do this. They need to know it is more than just a diet issue—it's a health issue. It is about becoming, and remaining, a fit, healthy, well-fed person—in control of your life and your diet.

Setting Some Ground Rules

Visual cues are a major influence on why we are drawn to certain foods. We literally eat with our eyes. So going about one's business in a home that has food on display can be dangerous. If there are foods that you decide you need to have around the house for others, but that you find potential triggers, keep in mind the old saying "out of sight, out of mind" and establish some new habits.

- *Make it inconvenient.* Keep foods, packages, cookie jars, and other containers off the kitchen counter. Also keep them off convenient or easy-to-reach shelves. The prospect of pulling out and climbing up onto the stepladder to reach a bag of potato chips nestled on the top shelf may be enough on some occasions to make you say, "Oh, forget about it."
- *Establish junk-free zones.* You can designate certain areas free and clear of junk food or other triggers: e.g., your house, the car, the patio. Don't forbid foods, but forbid them from those areas of your life. Junk-free zones, a.k.a. trigger-free zones, show what foods are important to you and why, while at the same time allowing your kids, your mate, or your roommate some control or autonomy in their own lives.
- *Take it outside.* If someone insists on buying Häagen-Dazs, just ask them either to do it when you aren't around or to do it somewhere else. If the kids must have a slice of pizza because their whole gang is getting one, fine, but keep it outside.

PEOPLE GAIN WEIGHT WITH THEIR FINGERS THAN WITH THEIR MOUTHS

- *Buy tea canisters.* Provide your children, maybe even your spouse, with individual tea canisters that they can keep in their closet or in some secret hiding place and in which they can store those special foods of theirs that may cause you problems. (They can keep the canisters anywhere as long as they're out of your reach.)
- *Lock it up.* If someone feels they just *have* to have access to their favorite treat at any time, give them their very own lockable cabinet or box where they can keep these foods. Then make use of the foolproof $7.95 solution—give them a lock and make sure you don't have access to the combination or key!

Many of my clients could have saved themselves the thousands of dollars they spent going to weight program after weight program by going to a locksmith instead. I grant you, many people think this is an extreme solution. *Don't worry about what's extreme.* Don't worry about what's normal. That is the preoccupation of the insecure. Life is short; do what works for *your* life. Worry more about reaching a normal weight than finding a normal way to store food.

I so admire Marissa, one of my female clients who was a top executive in the fashion industry. Marissa convinced her disbelieving husband to use a lockbox for his chips and nosh foods—she knew that they had been responsible for her falling off her diets in the past. These foods were just too tempting—and he insisted on having them available. Marissa is open-minded, flexible, and willing to do what works to be a winner. She went for the $7.95 solution.

The key to the lockbox, for some, may be the key to a new life of thin. Remember, behavior (even apparently silly behavior) speaks louder than words. You must teach your children, your spouse, and your friends around you something special through your behavior with food. You can no longer teach them habits that will cause great discomfort and chip away at the quality and length of their lives. It is time to teach better habits and a more modern set of values about food.

Going Shopping: Thin Starts in the Supermarket

You can't eat the right foods if you don't buy the right foods. I am often amazed when I see the amount of sugar-filled, fat-laden, processed, prepackaged, and nonnutritive foods I see piled in other shopping carts when I go to the store. If you keep these foods in the house—even under the pretext of having them for company or the kids—you are setting yourself up for disaster. For most people—particularly women—the most dangerous area in the world is their own kitchen.

The most basic rule of shopping in the Food Control Training Plan is: *If you don't buy it, you won't eat it.* When shopping, ask yourself, "Do I have a history of abusing this type of food?" If you do, don't buy it.

You don't need the finger foods and junk foods that may once have filled your pantry and refrigerator, and neither do your family or guests! If you care about people, why would you serve them foods you know are unhealthy? Why would you feed them something that will raise their cholesterol level and clog their arteries? Why would you put before them foods that might prompt them to lose control of their eating and become as enslaved by food as you once were?

There is no excuse for having trigger foods—or any kind of junk food—in your home. You can stock your larder and refrigerator with plenty of healthy foods that are easy to prepare, fun to eat, and far more delicious than the junk most food advertisers would have you believe you cannot live without. To help you along the way, I have developed (with considerable help from my clients!) the Ten Commandments of Dieting.

Commandment 1: Don't shop hungry. Most people make poor food choices when they shop because they are shopping with their taste buds. They shop when they are hungry and end up easy prey for the clever packaging and triggering power of the junk foods that line supermarket shelves. So protect yourself. Always eat something—if only a piece of fruit—before you go to the supermarket. Avoid shopping in the late afternoon when blood sugar tends to drop. The best time to shop is in the morning after breakfast.

Commandment 2: Make a list. The simplest trick for avoiding shopping triggers is to know what you are shopping for. Take time before you go to the store to make out a list of precisely what you need to buy. Plan out some of the meals you want to have in the coming days and make sure you have all the ingredients you'll need. Think in terms of actual meals rather than quick snacks and remember—something as simple as a cup of soup and a sandwich can qualify as a meal, too.

Commandment 3: Stay out of the junk food aisle. Most supermarkets have very kindly grouped all the worst trigger and junk foods together—in one bright, seductive, and very dangerous aisle. Stay out of it. There is nothing you need there.

Commandment 4: Read labels. The U.S. Food and Drug Administration now requires all food manufacturers to provide detailed nutritional information on all products. Use it. Look at the label to find out how many calories from fat the food contains and how many of its carbohydrates are in the form of sugar. Any food with more than 25 percent of its calories from fat should be avoided and any food that is high in sugars should also be kept out of your cart.

Commandment 5: Avoid processing. In general, the more processed a food is, the fewer nutrients it has and the more additives (like sugar and salt) it contains. A canned pear is not the same as a fresh one. So stock up on fresh items whenever possible. When you do buy canned or frozen vegetables, beans, soups, and so on, always read the labels carefully to avoid hidden fat, salt, and sugars.

Commandment 6: Don't shop as if stocking an air raid shelter. The average American pantry and refrigerator usually contain enough food to feed a small army for a couple of months or longer. This may be the most clear evidence of our immigrant "food is good" mind set. Even though there are all-night supermarkets dotting the landscape, we still shop as though famine were just around the corner. Keeping a supply of healthy staples will make your life easier and help you in gaining control. Stop by the store every three days or so to get fresh vegetables and fruits. Believe me, the supermarket is not going to disappear overnight and there are plenty of other things you can do with the space now occupied by three dozen cans of franks and beans.

Commandment 7: Avoid hydrogenated fats. For years, food oil companies have been telling us that margarines made from hydrogenated vegetable oils are heart-healthy alternatives to products high in saturated fats (like butter and lard). We now know this isn't so. Hydrogenation—the chemical process that turns a liquid oil into semisolid margarine—changes the shape of the fat molecule into something the human body cannot recognize or use. As a result, these *trans* fats actually end up causing many of the same problems as saturated fats. So avoid margarines and any processed food that lists hydrogenated or partially hydrogenated vegetable oils among its ingredients. Instead, go for one of the newer spreads that does not contain *trans* fats, or try fruit and vegetable spreads (see pages 179, 299).

Commandment 8: *Avoid tropical oils.* Certain oils from tropical plants—most notably palm and coconut oils—are very high in saturated fat, even if they have no cholesterol. Indeed, all plant oils are cholesterol-free and some unscrupulous food companies have taken advantage of this fact to advertise their products as cholesterol-free even when they contain lots of saturated fats.

Commandment 9: *Avoid added sugars.* Sugar is everywhere under many names. In fact, ounce for ounce, ketchup gets more of its calories from sugar than ice cream does. Even if you are cutting back on sugar at the table, you could still be getting it in your processed foods, so keep an eye out for any of the "oses"—sucrose, lactose, maltose, galactose, fructose—as well as the various other pseudonyms for highly refined sugars—corn syrup, high fructose corn syrup, mannitol, honey, maple sugar, and so on.

Commandment 10: *Buy single-serving packages.* If you are going to keep snack foods (such as low-fat popcorn or pretzels) in the house, make sure you buy single-serving packages that will help you limit intake. Big, bargain-sized bags are an invitation to uncontrolled eating. It may cost a little more, but loss of control will cost you a lot more. Remember, calories cost more than dollars—you have to wear them.

Spreading the Word

If you love (or at least care for) the people you live with, you will probably want to introduce them to the satisfaction—both emotional and culinary—of Food Control Training. After all, if it improves your weight, your health, and your well-being, you are bound to want to spread the word. Ex-foodies, like ex-smokers, can often be very evangelical.

If you feel yourself being struck with missionary zeal, more power to you. But accept this one warning—don't preach! In fact, if you really want to win your friends and loved ones over to a more healthful diet, the best thing you can do is become a silent food lobbyist, an advocate for food control who gets the message across without beating others over the head with it. Try following these four simple rules.

1. *Don't nag.* Don't harangue those around you with constant talk of food control. Don't make them feel paranoid or uncomfortable about what they eat. Let your weight loss and happiness speak for you. As Dr. Dean Ornish has said, most people "want to feel free. And you can't feel free if someone is telling you to do something, even if it is supposedly for your own good. That goes back to Adam and Eve, when God said, 'Don't eat the apple.' We saw how effective that was—and that was God talking."

2. *Be subtle.* An effective food lobbyist respects the rights of others to live as they choose but at the same time protects his or her own. You will find that in protecting yourself from certain trigger foods or situations, others will benefit as well. So how do you lobby in a food-smart way? Be creative when it comes to social events: Don't always go to the same restaurant with the same fat-filled menu. Encourage your partner or friends to try another establishment where everyone can eat in a healthful way. Or meet a friend at a museum or a local park instead of at a restaurant. At dinner parties, if you or your partner is a Prowler or a Picker, avoid the early phase—when the hors d'oeuvres are most plentiful. Teach your partner some of the defensive measures discussed earlier, such as pouring a glass of tomato juice for each of you so that you won't be hungry—and thus vulnerable—when you arrive at the event.

3. *"If you serve it, they will eat."* People will go for what you put in front of them, so make sure that what's there is good—healthy, tasty, and satisfying. Serve healthy snack alternatives—nonfat frozen yogurt instead of ice cream, diet iced tea instead of regular, or an Interior Design Nutritionals' Fiberry snack bar (at only 80 calories) instead of the usual fatty granola bar. (Many of my clients have discovered a host of Interior Design products, made by Nu Skin, that are both healthful *and* satisfying. They even got me hooked—one of my favorites is their Appeal Shake. You can order Nu Skin products by calling 800-487-1500.)

4. *Never tell them what you're serving.* If they eat it and it tastes good, that's all that matters. Buy what you need and what you know is a food-smart purchase, and don't tell your spouse or houseguests that a particular food is low fat

---

or diet. Let them enjoy it. Don't make it an issue when it doesn't need to be one.

If, after all this, your friends or family claim that they are too old to change, don't buy it. It's never too late for change, especially food control.

For those readers who have a spouse, child, friend, or loved one with health and weight issues, these subtle maneuvers will do more to assist them than all the nagging, threats, arguments, and ultimatums in the world. And since we are all visual eaters, if you stock your kitchen with healthful alternatives, the visual eaters in your home won't be able to stop themselves—they'll have to eat healthy. And I'll wager that they'll have to admit they like it.

But What About the Children?

Children learn by what they live. Many households are teaching children the very same foodie beliefs and habits that led to the parents' weight problems. If you want your children to escape the foodie trap and live long, healthy lives, you must be their instructor. You must teach them more than what most of us learned from our parents.

We are learning that more and more children are falling prey to supposedly adult maladies such as arteriosclerosis. And it's not just clogged arteries. Atherosclerotic lesions have been discovered in both the aorta and the coronary arteries in people below the age of twenty. The noted Bogalusa Heart Study, which tracks the heart health of children in the Bogalusa, Louisiana, area, has actually found the earliest stages of heart disease in scores of youngsters, some as young as three years old!

Childhood obesity is a tremendous problem that has been increasing exponentially for years. High blood pressure affects 1 to 2 percent of children. And the numbers only get worse: By the time the kids are in their teens and early twenties, some 20 percent may fall prey to the disease.

The future for these couch potato kids will prove to be increasingly grim unless we start changing our presumptions about what kids expect and by what influences they can truly be victimized. Living in a house without Ho-Hos hardly seems as terrible a burden as we sometimes make it out to be.

Children need to be exposed to a set of healthy values regarding foods even as we limit their exposure to the foods and habits that contribute to overweight. Limiting exposure and availability, after all, is quite different from forbidding certain foods. When the children get older, *they* can decide how much TV or junk food to consume; then their decisions will be based on the health information we've given them, not the old "food as reward" response from our own childhoods.

In the many junk food–free homes that *do* exist out there, kids don't rebel or object. They don't feel diminished or deprived. Because they have been raised without foodie expectations and beliefs, they are free of the food obsessions that afflict so many adults. And because they have not been inundated with the tastes and textures of these foods, they are also free of the cravings and taste for these foods.

If you are a parent, you can give your children this same legacy of freedom. It is easier when children are younger, of course, but even older children can be weaned away from less than healthy foods and food habits. Here are two ways to meet that goal.

Set a regular dinner hour. This can be difficult, especially in dual-earner households with hectic work schedules, but it's worth the effort. Too often parents of obese children focus on how much they eat, whereas many researchers today believe that *what* a child is eating may be more significant—and there's no better way to know than to be there to watch. Set the dinner hour and a snack time (like right after school), and stick to them. Make sure you know what your children take to school for lunch or ask what they buy at the school cafeteria. Continue monitoring so you always have a good idea of their daily menu.

Children thrive on a structured environment and it is no different when it comes to eating. You may find that setting out a nutritious meal after years of unhealthy dinners may go unappreciated and your child may still refuse to eat any of his green beans. That's okay, as long as you don't let him negotiate some other food instead. The more nutritionally varied his meals are, the more the child will have to choose from and the more likely, as time passes, he will grow to enjoy and prefer the food choices his parents present to him.

Don't be a Spartan. Kids will be kids, and that means they may pig out at a birthday party or class field trip. As long as you continue to offer your child healthful and good-tasting meals, he will appreciate the benefits of smart eating. Bubblegum, cupcakes, and the occasional brownie can all have a place in childhood as long as these pig-out sessions don't become increasingly frequent behaviors and are not used for solace or reward.

How to Entertain Safely

Whether hosting a blowout party with wall-to-wall people or conducting a more intimate gathering of a few relatives or friends, entertaining is sure to pose troubles for anyone who is trying to control a weight problem.

First, the house is packed with food, sometimes days or weeks ahead of time. The easy availability of a variety of trigger foods would be a tough match for anyone, let alone an individual who may still be frequently prone to slipups. Second, your stress level is higher than normal. Even the most informal of get-togethers with the best of friends can be an anxiety-ridden experience for the conscientious host who is worried about making sure everybody is comfortable and has what they need, not to mention whether there is enough ice, whether the coffeemaker is on the fritz again, and what to do if you're planning to sit outdoors and it rains. And third, what happens all too often at the end of the evening is the company leaves and the food stays. There are often huge amounts of leftovers to be collected, wrapped up, and stored away—a very dangerous situation. If you are food-smart, however, you should be able to overcome each of these hurdles.

When buying food for company, there's often no way around buying items that you wouldn't ordinarily bring into your home, whether it is something specific for a houseguest or foods for a particular holiday. When this is the case, you need to treat the occasion as an isolated incident. Buy only the exact number or amount of a food item that you need and, if possible, try to make those purchases only a day or two in advance. Store the dangerous trigger foods out of sight until cooked or served.

When planning and hosting the party, try to keep it simple and do everything you can ahead of time in order to keep your worrying to a minimum. If you are a stress eater, you have got to work especially hard to calm down. Look back to our discussion of stress eating in the first step of food control, your Eating Print. Review the advice on what to think so your immediate response to the stress won't be turning to food. Pull out your food control tapes and listen to a few the days preceding and the day of the event. And, if all else fails, pay close attention to yourself near the end of the party and don't succumb to picking at the leftovers.

Women especially must watch out for the last fifteen minutes of any party or get-together in their home. These times are toughest because an excessive amount of food is in view. Try to make sure that you clean up as much as possible before the last few stragglers leave you alone with a pile of leftover triggers. People always offer to help clear; accept that favor. Or make clearing one of your children's weekly chores. If there are any special foods bought in honor of a houseguest, they should get going when the guests do, as should your trigger foods. Any way you can, the sooner you get these foods put away or out of your house, the better.

I don't like to label any food as "good" or "bad" per se. It is better to distinguish between foods that are good for you and your individual needs and those that are bad for you. You need to make a distinction between those foods in your life. You don't want to throw out good-for-you foods. Store or freeze any leftovers that are on your eating plan. As for fat-, calorie-, or salt-laden leftovers, do not hesitate— use the garbage pail, disposal, or trash compactor immediately. I know, people hate throwing food away. "It's wasteful," I've been told. Or "It's not environmentally correct." Yet is it not a greater waste to throw out your health and your clothes?

I can't tell you how many of my clients had trouble with that concept at first. Perhaps they are reminded of the starving children in the world. Perhaps they feel it somehow a selfish and careless act. This is another case of value confusion—being protective about food is not nearly as important as being protective about your health and control. To throw out food you have a long history of abusing or leftovers you know will go into your stomach if they don't go into the garbage pail is not an act of selfishness. It is not an act of wastefulness, but one of self-acceptance. Is it selfish or wasteful for a person who wants to quit smoking to crumple up a pack of cigarettes and toss it in the trash? On the contrary, those who cared for that person's health would applaud such an action. The wrong foods can be just as devastating to a life as nicotine.

AFTER A BASH

For bigger festivities, with more leftover food than you can cope with, I suggest trying alternatives like City Harvest, a national organization that comes to your door, carts away your leftovers, and distributes them to various shelters and social service organizations. Check your local white or Yellow Pages for any national, state, and local relief organizations that can help others with your leftovers while protecting you from them.

The foods I am suggesting you toss out are not vital foods. I'm telling you to toss out pounds of sugar and globs of fat. The starving children of the world don't need sugary cereals, puffed snacks, stale cake, and the other valueless foods we obsess over. They need *real food*—wheat and milk and fresh drinking water. They need the basics.

So do you. So make room in your cabinets and your refrigerator for the basics, the good foods of life. And you'll find that you're not wasting a thing.

When Your Weight Loss Threatens *Their* Peace of Mind

As much as the people around you may be thrilled by the new, slim, healthy you, they can also be a bit taken aback and even intimidated. If you've been heavy for many years, the new thin you can seem like a stranger. If you were once thin but gained weight over the years, your partner may have gotten used to this change, even if he or she is not *happy* with it.

Back when you were too heavy and too easily winded to exert yourself with the kids, did your husband take on the task of playing tag or teaching the kids to ride bikes? Now that you're healthy enough to do a little running and bike riding yourself, he may feel a bit as if his territory has been invaded. Was your wife's pet project always trying to get you to lose weight? Or did she get used to playing the martyr, the one her friends quietly pitied because they felt she deserved a better-looking mate? Well, what is she going to do now that you've dropped 50 pounds and suddenly *you're* the one getting all the compliments and admiring glances when the two of you walk into a room?

The balance of power changes when weight changes, and couples and friends and family must be prepared for that. Even the most supportive friend, family member, or mate may find him- or herself subtly trying to undermine your weight-control efforts to restore the status quo. Dealing with such subtle, often unconscious sabotage is important, both for your health and the health of your relationships.

Sometimes the sabotage will come in the form of forgetting which foods you'd like kept out of the house or accidentally leaving your trigger foods around in plain sight. At other times, it may take the form of unwarranted criticisms—you've gotten vain, your avoidance of triggers means you're weak, you looked better with a little more meat on your bones, and so on. On occasion it may even be outright anger—"You're different now that you've lost weight!" Whatever the form, confront the sabotage for what it is. Don't go on the attack, but let the person know how it makes you feel. Keep the lines of communication open. Living thin requires making many adjustments—not only on your part but on the part of the people around you. Be patient, be honest, and be communicative and you can all arrive at a new and healthy status quo.

LIVING THIN . . . FOREVER

We are standing on the brink of a new world as surely as our forebears did when they heard the first mechanized roars of the Industrial Revolution. The world was never the same after that. And just as our eating habits and the kinds of foods we ate changed at that point in history, so, too, can our eating and our knowledge of food today take a new direction.

You may have bought this book because you wanted a weight book. You may have read it because of its diet. But in the end, this book—and living thin itself—is not really about dieting or weight. Rather, it is about self-mastery. Living thin is a philosophy of life in which you—not food—are in control, a philosophy that allows you to rise above the programming of the unenlightened but well-meaning generations that have come before.

Our parents and grandparents had an excuse. They did not know that the foods they associated with wealth and prosperity would eventually cut short our lives and increase our risk of diabetes, cancer, heart disease, and a host of other maladies. But we know better, and with that knowledge comes responsibility—a responsibility to judge food not by the ancient standards of taste, texture, and aesthetics alone but looking at the total mosaic, how it affects our lives as a whole. Our ancestors thought it was our destiny to be fat and the way they were taught to eat and cook assured that such a fate was indeed the only way. They had no alternatives.

But we do.

A cultural shift has already started to take place. Just look at the new and ever more impressive medical discoveries and nutritional research. Never before have we been more informed.

Just look at the proliferation of gyms, health clubs, aerobics studios, and personal trainers (totally unheard of in our ancestors' generations); at the phantasmagorical array of gourmet foods in supermarkets, so many low in fat, calories, preservatives, and higher than ever before in taste and freshness; at the number of restaurants expanding their menus, adding new "lite" items and salads that make you think of anything but mere lettuce. Even the fast-food establishments are falling in line.

Look at the cookbooks that only thirty years ago were full of killer recipes that spared not a drop of butter, oil, or fat of any kind. Red meat was a given. Today, many cookbooks have become food-smart, emphasizing heart-healthy cooking tips. Look at the new federal labeling requirements that have made food packaging more truthful and infinitely easier to read.

Slowly but surely, our cultural consciousness is catching up to our biological reality. Part of living as a complete human being is to have respect for your body and your own life history. This is what is meant by "Know thyself"; it is the essence of self-understanding. The recent decades of prosperity and scientific advancement have provided us with the opportunity to know ourselves and to develop a new, healthy mind-set wherein food is a part of life, enhancing life, not the centerpiece that diminishes it.

With the strategies and eating plan presented in this

book, you can do just that. You can attain the mind-set that leads to a trim, toned, triumphant look. You can join the winners at weight loss who have mastered the skills that not only extend their *life span* but revitalize their *health span* and *youth span.*

There has never been a better time to succeed at getting healthy. And you can get there with Food Control Training.

To age well is not an accident. It is a gift that those who care can give to themselves. It is a process of stepping back from the old cultural programming, realizing that you cannot eat it all as you age and still be thin. This is not the principle of a weight-loss program—this is a principle of reality and the key to life enhancement. True success at weight loss is that simple.

You can and will age well. You have learned to treat your calories like dollars. You have accepted that your body, like your checkbook, has a budget and that that budget changes over time. You know that becoming thin, staying thin, and living thin is not about luck but is a learned skill that grows and becomes easier over time, allowing you to become a stronger, more resilient human being.

You are on your way to breaking out of the backward value system that spawns the deprivation mind-set. You know that, for most of us, thin is not a birthright, nor is being able to have anything you want any time you want. Finally, you are able to overcome the fear and immobility conjured up by deprivation and cravings. You are getting beyond the food whining, beyond your concerns about a lack of willpower, for now you see it is not about willpower but focus and control. Now you truly see that, in the final analysis, it is not at all about deprivation but liberation!

Each day, when I walk home from my office, though the hour may be late, I don't feel at all fatigued, for the people

I have seen during that day, and their victories, have not drained my strength but renewed it. In the end, I have never considered my work to be about dieting or weight control but about giving my clients the ability to rewrite the script for the rest of their lives and to end the chapters of pain, disappointment, and suffering that their weight problem has brought. This work is about pushing forward the boundaries of human freedom in your life.

Some people are given the opportunity to paint on a canvas. I have been given the opportunity to paint on the canvas of human life, to be part of a creative process that leads to a brighter future for the individuals I work with at my office and through the pages of this book. Part of this future making involves overcoming your self-doubts and realizing that the greatest weight you carry is not the pounds but the failures and setbacks of the past. *Thin Tastes Better* turns these setbacks into lessons. This book is the classroom where you learn a new way of living and thinking.

This will prove to be one of the most creative things you will do in your adult life. It is very rare in the course of living that such a moment comes along, that by making just a few changes, you can alter the quality and character of every single day of the rest of your life—even the length of that life itself. Like a smart, lucrative investment, you will receive a payback every day, or should I say every morning, as you look in that mirror when you get dressed. I wish you the very best in discovering that for yourself. Everyone deserves such thrilling discoveries.

Today, right now, after you put down this book, you have the opportunity to rediscover yourself as a thin person, as a healthy person, the master of your own destiny. You have a chance to see that thin *can* last a lifetime, along with all the rewards that thin brings. Not only that, you have the opportunity to make changes that will influence generations to come.

You may have failed many times in the past and doubt whether you can follow a script for a new life. But believe me: Each person who started my program felt the same way on the first day. But with one step, one day, one containment, one victory at a time, they became wiser and more confident of the next. Yes, it does take some work, but never as much work as *not* doing it. For not doing it is much harder. In life, we sometimes forget that inaction can cost much more than taking action and solving a problem.

This is your opportunity to be a winner. Take it.

MENUS, RECIPES,
AND RESOURCES

A WEEK OF SAMPLE MENUS

You will find here a week's worth of sample menus to show you that the Food Control Eating Plan can mean delectable meals.

DAY ONE

BREAKFAST
1 Special K Fat Free Waffle (2 for men) with 2 tablespoons *Fresh Fruit Compote* (page 288)
$1/2$ grapefruit
coffee or tea

LUNCH
Salad Niçoise (page 281)
1 cup *Blender Gazpacho* (page 259)
flavored seltzer or diet soda

DINNER
Poached Fish with Vegetables (page 264)
Green Beans with Sautéed Mushrooms (page 275)
mixed green salad
flavored seltzer or diet soda
Poached Apples and Pears with Berry Sauce (page 287)

DAY TWO

BREAKFAST
1 poached egg
1 *Complementary Light and Airy Muffin* (page 292) or 1 slice toasted protein bread with 1 teaspoon all-fruit preserves or 1 pat of margarine
coffee or tea

LUNCH
Grilled Vegetable Plate (page 276)
diet soda or flavored seltzer

DINNER
Herbed Chicken Breasts (page 263)

Steamed Asparagus with Sun-Dried Tomato Sauce (page 280)
mixed green salad
baked potato
Fruit Smoothies (page 290)

DAY THREE

BREAKFAST 8 ounces plain low-fat yogurt with 2 tablespoons Grape-Nuts and
1 small banana or 1 cup berries
coffee or tea
LUNCH large bowl *Broccoli Soup* (page 258)
mixed green salad
flavored seltzer or diet soda
DINNER *Scallops with White Wine and Lemon* (page 267)
baked sweet potato
Roasted Vegetable Kabobs (page 272)
mixed green salad
glass of wine

DAY FOUR

BREAKFAST poached or scrambled egg
1 slice toasted diet or protein bread with 1 teaspoon all-fruit preserves
coffee or tea
LUNCH *Grilled Chicken Salad* (page 260)
flavored seltzer or diet soda
DINNER *Braised Fish with Artichoke Hearts and Red Peppers* (page 265)
baked potato
mixed green salad
1 slice *Fresh Fruit Pie with Nut Crust* (page 289)

DAY FIVE

BREAKFAST Egg-white omelette stuffed with *Ratatouille* (page 278)

1 *Complementary Light and Airy Muffin* (page 292) with 1 tea-
    spoon all-fruit preserves
coffee or tea

LUNCH   *White Bean and Tuna Salad* (page 282) on bed of red leaf lettuce
flavored seltzer or diet soda

DINNER   *Herbed Turkey Burgers* (page 262)
Potato-Basil Crisp (page 277)
mixed green salad
4 ounces fat-free vanilla yogurt with $1/4$ cup *Fresh Fruit Compote*
    (page 288)

DAY SIX

BREAKFAST   1 *Mayor's Muffin* (page 291), toasted
2 slices reduced-fat cheese
$1/4$ cantaloupe
coffee or tea

LUNCH   large bowl of *Blender Gazpacho* (page 259)
mixed green salad
flavored seltzer or diet soda

DINNER   *Garlic Shrimp* (page 266) over *Spaghetti Squash* (page 270) with
    Low-Fat Tomato Sauce (page 284)
Banana Cream (page 286)

DAY SEVEN

BREAKFAST   cold cereal with skim milk and 1 small banana or $1/2$ cup berries
coffee or tea

LUNCH   *Ratatouille* (page 278) over baked potato
flavored seltzer or diet soda

DINNER   *Vegetable Lasagna* (page 268)
mixed green salad
glass of wine

RECIPES FOR THIN

Cooking for thin is really fairly easy even without specific recipes, but this selection of stocks and salads, and vegetable, dessert, dressing, and main-dish recipes, will give you a head start. These recipes are culled from several of the cookbooks recommended on page 309, as well as from the kitchens of my clients and chef Susan Knightly. (Note: A minimal amount of olive oil is included as an ingredient in some recipes, assuming you are using a regular cast-iron skillet or stainless steel pan. If you have nonstick pans, you can cut the amount of olive oil in half or, in some cases, eliminate it entirely.) Enjoy!

STOCKS

One-Pot Chicken and Stock
Makes 2 to 3 quarts of broth
A chicken, some water, and a few spices and vegetables make a delicious low-fat broth *and* provide lots of tender chicken meat for sandwiches, salads, or quick hot meals.

1 3- to 5-pound chicken
1/4 teaspoon dried sage
2 small onions, peeled and quartered
4 garlic cloves
1 celery stalk, chopped
1 carrot, chopped
1/2 teaspoon salt
1/2 teaspoon black pepper
1/2 teaspoon dried thyme
1 teaspoon dried parsley or 3 sprigs, chopped
1 bay leaf

1. Rinse the chicken. Rub half the sage into the bird's cavity and half on the skin.
2. Stuff the cavity with 1 onion, the garlic, and half the celery and carrot.
3. Place the chicken in a heavy stockpot with the remaining onion, celery, carrot, spices, and herbs. Cover the chicken with water and bring to a boil. Reduce the heat to low and simmer for 2 hours.
4. Remove the chicken and strain the broth. Let the broth sit until tepid.
5. While the broth cools, remove the chicken meat from the bones. (Be thorough!) The meat can be refrigerated in an airtight container for up to 3 days.
6. When the broth has cooled, spoon off the congealed fat. Use the broth within 4 days or freeze it in jars and use as necessary.

Simple Vegetable Stock
Makes about 1½ quarts

Vegetable stock is a multipurpose liquid that can be used as a base for soups and sauces as well as a cooking tool. Although almost any vegetable can be used for stock, cruciferous vegetables (broccoli, cabbage, cauliflower, and their relatives) should be avoided, since their distinctive flavors can overwhelm a stock.

1 onion, finely chopped	*3 sprigs parsley*
2 carrots, chopped	*1 bay leaf*
2 celery stalks, chopped	*1 tablespoon chopped fresh*
3 cups raw vegetables	*thyme or 1 teaspoon dried*
1 tablespoon vegetable oil	*2 whole cloves*
(preferably canola or olive)	*2 garlic cloves*

1. Rinse and peel all the vegetables. (If you're using organic produce, just rinse.)
2. In a large pot, heat the oil. Quickly add the onion and cook until light brown, stirring occasionally. Add the remainder of the ingredients and cover. Cook 10 minutes on low heat.
3. Cover with 2 quarts of water, bring to a boil, reduce the heat, and simmer 1½ hours. Strain the stock and use immediately or refrigerate for future use. If a more intense flavor is desired, return the strained stock to the stove and reduce the liquid by half.

Soups

Broccoli Soup
Serves 6
At only 24 calories a cup, this soup is a nutrient-rich, satisfying alternative to creamed soups.

2 tablespoons vegetable oil
1 onion, peeled and finely chopped
3 garlic cloves, peeled and chopped
1 teaspoon dried marjoram or 1 tablespoon fresh
1 teaspoon dried thyme
1/8 teaspoon nutmeg
2 celery stalks, finely chopped
2 scallions, trimmed and coarsely chopped

1 1/2 pounds broccoli, washed and separated into florets and stems
6 cups vegetable stock or water
2 tablespoons minced fresh dill
Salt
Black pepper

1. Warm the oil in a large stockpot over medium heat. (Don't let the oil get so hot that it smokes.) Add the onion and cook until it is translucent, then add the garlic, marjoram, thyme, and nutmeg. Sauté 3 minutes. Add the celery and scallions and cook 5 minutes. Add the broccoli stems and the stock, cover, and simmer 30 minutes.
2. Add the broccoli florets and cook 2 minutes. Remove from the heat and blend in a food processor or blender, adding the dill as it's blending. Season with salt and pepper and serve.

Blender Gazpacho

Serves 6 to 8

Gazpacho is the ultimate summer soup—easy to make, easy to store, and delicious served chilled right from the refrigerator.

1½ pounds ripe tomatoes, peeled (6 to 7)

3 to 4 cups tomato juice or 1 22-ounce can plum tomatoes and 6 ounces tomato juice

2 garlic cloves, peeled

1 small onion, chopped

1 small cucumber, peeled and coarsely chopped

1 carrot, coarsely chopped

1 green pepper, seeded and coarsely chopped

2 parsley sprigs, coarsely chopped

4 tablespoons chopped fresh basil

Juice of 1 lemon

Salt and black pepper, to taste

1. Submerge tomatoes in boiling water for 1 minute; remove and peel.
2. Blend together all the ingredients in a blender until smooth.
3. Chill for several hours if possible. Adjust the seasonings to taste. (The soup will keep in the refrigerator for 2 to 3 days.)

POULTRY

Grilled Chicken Salad

Serves 4

A mix of crisp grilled chicken, greens, potatoes, and a light herb dressing, this salad is a meal in itself.

2 boneless chicken breasts

MARINADE

2 tablespoons olive oil
2 tablespoons balsamic vinegar
1 bay leaf
1/2 teaspoon dried rosemary

1/2 teaspoon dried thyme
1 garlic clove, minced
1/4 teaspoon salt
Dash of black pepper

DRESSING

2 tablespoons extra virgin olive oil
2 tablespoons canola oil
1/4 cup vegetable or chicken stock
3 tablespoons vinegar

2 garlic cloves, minced
1 teaspoon minced parsley
1/2 teaspoon dried thyme
1/2 teaspoon paprika
Salt
Black pepper

SALAD

2 medium red potatoes, rinsed and quartered
1/2 cup green beans, rinsed, trimmed, and halved
1 carrot, peeled and thinly sliced into 1-inch slices
1/2 cup mixed vegetables (broccoli and cauliflower

florets, snow peas, 1-inch slices of zucchini)
1 head green leaf lettuce, rinsed, cored, and cut into thin strips
2 medium tomatoes, quartered
1 red pepper, cored, seeded, and thinly sliced

1. Prepare the grill or preheat the broiler.
2. Slice the chicken breasts in half lengthwise. In a bowl, combine the marinade ingredients and whisk well. Add the chicken and marinate for at least 15 minutes.
3. In a small bowl, whisk together the dressing ingredients. Set aside.
4. Fill a small pot with water and bring to a boil. Add the potatoes and cook for 10 to 15 minutes, or until a fork easily pierces the potato. Drain and rinse in cold water.
5. Fill a medium pot with water. Bring to a boil and add the green beans, carrot, and mixed vegetables. Cook for no more than 2 minutes, then immediately drain and rinse the vegetables with cold water.
6. Remove the chicken from the marinade and discard the marinade. Place the chicken on the grill or under the broiler for 4 minutes per side. The cooking time will vary depending on the thickness of the breast. After 8 minutes, check the chicken by piercing it with a sharp knife. The juices should run clear when done. Remove from the heat, let cool a few minutes, then slice into thin strips.
7. In a large bowl, toss the lettuce, tomatoes, and red pepper. Add the beans, carrot, mixed vegetables, and potatoes and toss lightly. Add the chicken and dressing and toss well. Serve on chilled salad plates.

Herbed Turkey Burgers

Serves 4 to 6

Ground white meat turkey is an excellent low-fat alternative to ground beef. However, prepackaged ground poultry often contains ground-up skin and fat, so buy your own fresh turkey breast and have the meat department grind it for you.

1½ pounds ground raw turkey	*1 tablespoon dried basil*
1 egg	*2 garlic cloves, minced*
3 tablespoons soy sauce	*¼ teaspoon black pepper*
1 tablespoon dried marjoram	

1. Preheat the broiler.
2. Combine the turkey, egg, soy sauce, marjoram, basil, garlic, and black pepper. Form into 4 to 6 patties.
3. Broil the burgers until well done, about 10 minutes, turning once during cooking. Do not undercook.
4. Serve on toasted protein or diet bread, topped with a slice of no-fat cheese, horseradish, or salsa, alongside a mixed green salad.

Herbed Chicken Breasts
Serves 4

3 tablespoons olive oil
2 teaspoons prepared mustard
  (Dijon or Pommery)
2 teaspoons water
1 garlic clove, minced
$1/4$ teaspoon ground cumin
$1/2$ teaspoon paprika

$1/2$ teaspoon dried thyme or
  $1^1/2$ teaspoons fresh
$1/2$ teaspoon chopped parsley
$1/2$ teaspoon salt
Black pepper
4 chicken breast halves, skin
  removed

1. Preheat the broiler. Combine the oil, mustard, water, garlic, spices, herbs, salt, and pepper in a small bowl.
2. Place the chicken on a baking sheet and brush both sides with half of the oil-herb mixture. Broil the chicken, bone side up, for 10 minutes. Turn and brush all but 2 tablespoons of the remaining mixture on top of the breasts and cook 7 minutes, or until the chicken juices run clear when the breast is pierced with a fork. Brush the remaining mixture on the chicken for a moistened look. Remove and serve.

FISH

Poached Fish with Vegetables
Serves 4

2 medium onions, sliced	*1/2* teaspoon dried rosemary
2 leeks, rinsed well and sliced	*1/2* teaspoon ground allspice
2 carrots, thinly sliced	2 teaspoons salt
2 celery stalks, sliced	2 tablespoons black pepper
1/2 cup chopped fresh dill	1 cup apple cider vinegar
1 tablespoon finely chopped parsley	4 4- to 6-ounce fish fillets (whitefish, cod, halibut, or salmon)
2 bay leaves	
1 teaspoon dried thyme	

1. Place all the vegetables, herbs, and spices in a large pot, cover, and let sit over very low heat for 5 minutes. After a minute or two, stir to prevent sticking and add a little water (this will combine and release the flavors of the vegetables and herbs).
2. Add the vinegar and 5 cups water, cover, and simmer for 12 minutes.
3. Add the fish and cook over medium-low heat until the fish is flaky and solid white (or pink, if salmon), usually 10 minutes per 1-inch-thick piece. Using a spatula, remove each fillet to a large bowl. Remove the bay leaves and divide the vegetables and stock among the bowls.

Braised Fish with Artichoke Hearts and Red Peppers

Serves 4 to 6

3 tablespoons olive oil
1 cup thinly sliced onions
1 red bell pepper, thinly sliced
   lengthwise
1 14-ounce can artichoke
   hearts, drained and
   quartered
1 teaspoon paprika

1 tablespoon chopped fresh
   dill
2 tablespoons chopped parsley
$3/4$ cup dry white wine or
   vermouth
$1^{1}/_2$ pounds firm fish fillets
Salt and black pepper

1. In a large skillet, heat the olive oil and sauté the onions for 3 minutes. Add the bell pepper and sauté for 3 more minutes.
2. Add the artichoke hearts, paprika, dill, and parsley. Sauté for 1 minute, stirring to prevent sticking.
3. Add the wine and lay the fish fillets, skin side down, on top of the simmering vegetables. Sprinkle with salt and pepper, cover the skillet, and cook for 5 to 10 minutes on low heat, until the fish flakes easily with a fork.
4. Remove the fish with a slotted spatula or large spoon. Bring the remaining juices to a boil and stir while the liquid reduces, about 2 minutes. Pour the juices and vegetables over the fish and serve.

Baked Salmon Steaks

Serves 6

This elegant fish recipe is a snap to prepare and provides ample amounts of heart-healthy omega-3 fatty acids.

2 tablespoons olive oil	2 tablespoons finely chopped parsley
1 large onion, sliced	
3 garlic cloves, minced	1/2 teaspoon black pepper
2 lemons, sliced	1/2 teaspoon salt
1 bunch fresh dill, minced	4 3- to 4-ounce salmon steaks

1. Preheat the oven to 400°F.
2. In a bowl, combine the oil, onion, garlic, lemons, dill, parsley, pepper, and salt. Place half of this mixture in a long baking dish, place the salmon steaks on top, then sprinkle the remaining mixture on the fish. Bake 30 to 40 minutes, or until the fish is opaque all the way through.

Garlic Shrimp

Serves 4

These shrimp are delicious hot or cold. Serve as hors d'oeuvres, over pasta, as part of a green salad, or alongside a baked potato and a green vegetable.

3/4 pound medium shrimp	1 tablespoon freshly squeezed lemon juice
1 tablespoon olive oil	
6 to 8 garlic cloves, minced	1/2 teaspoon salt
1 tablespoon minced parsley	1/8 teaspoon black pepper

1. Rinse the shrimp and peel off the shells and tails. Devein the shrimp by making a small, shallow incision along the back of the shrimp, then pulling out the vein.

2. In a large skillet, warm the olive oil over medium heat. Add the garlic and cook 1 minute, stirring constantly. Add the shrimp and sauté so the shrimp cook evenly and do not stick to the bottom of the pan. After 3 minutes, add the parsley, lemon juice, salt, and pepper and cook 1 minute more.

Scallops with White Wine and Lemon
Serves 4
Quick and simple, this is one of the tastiest ways to prepare scallops.

1 pound scallops (bay or sea)	*1 tablespoon white wine or*
2 teaspoons olive oil	*dry white vermouth*
2 to 3 tablespoons fresh lemon	*1 tablespoon chopped fresh*
juice	*dill*
1 garlic clove, minced	*¹/₈ teaspoon black pepper*

1. Clean the scallops. (If using large scallops, pull off the hard nubbin attached to the side of the scallop and cut in half.) Soak the scallops briefly in a bowl of very cold water to rid them of sand. Refrigerate until just before use.
2. Brush a medium-sized skillet with the oil. Sauté the scallops over high heat until they are lightly browned, about 3 minutes. If the scallops release a large amount of liquid, drain it off before step 3.
3. Add the lemon juice, wine, and garlic and cook a few minutes more until the liquid reduces.
4. Add the dill and pepper and sauté quickly.
5. Serve over whole wheat pasta or brown rice (or with a baked potato) along with a mixed green salad.

VEGETABLES

Vegetable Lasagna
Serves 6 to 8

Lasagna is usually a fat-laden dish, but this vegetable version omits the cheese and is very low in fat and high in nutrition and flavor. It is also perfect for experimentation—try adding other vegetables to the mix or playing with the balance of spices.

4 tablespoons plus 2
  teaspoons olive oil
1 16-ounce package lasagna
  noodles
1 medium onion, diced
2 garlic cloves, finely chopped
2 green peppers, diced
2 celery stalks, diced
2 carrots, diced
1/4 cup chopped parsley
Red wine or dry white
  vermouth (optional)
1 28-ounce can crushed
  tomatoes

1 green zucchini, sliced
  (1/4-inch slices)
1 gold zucchini, sliced
  (1/4-inch slices)
1 cup cooked chopped spinach
  (frozen is okay)
1/2 pound chopped asparagus
1 teaspoon dried oregano
1 teaspoon dried basil
1/2 teaspoon dried thyme
Salt and black pepper, to taste

1. Preheat the oven to 350°F.
2. Fill a large pot with water and bring to a rolling boil. Add 1 teaspoon olive oil to the water and carefully place the lasagna noodles in the pot. Cook for 7 to 10 minutes, or until the noodles are al dente—softened but not mushy. Drain the noodles in a large colander (try not to break the noodles in the process!) and place the noodles under cold running water to rinse.

3. While the noodles are cooking, heat the 4 tablespoons oil in a large skillet. Add the onion and sauté until golden.

4. Add the garlic and sauté 2 minutes.

5. Add the peppers, celery, carrots, and parsley. Cover and cook over medium heat for 5 minutes. (If the vegetables are sticking to the skillet, add just a splash of red wine or dry white vermouth.)

6. Add the tomatoes, zucchini, spinach, asparagus, oregano, basil, thyme, salt, and pepper. Cook for 5 minutes more.

7. Brush a large baking pan with the remaining 1 teaspoon olive oil. Alternate layers of vegetables and lasagna noodles, ending with a layer of vegetables. Cover the pan with foil and cook for 25 to 30 minutes.

No-Fat "Fried" Zucchini Sticks
Serves 4

Deep-fried vegetables are often all but unrecognizable beneath layers of batter and grease. This no-fat version replaces the batter with a flavorful marinade, and roasts the zucchini to a crispy finish with a melt-in-your-mouth center. It works equally well with broccoli and cauliflower.

1 teaspoon olive oil
2 medium gold or green
  zucchini

MARINADE

¹/₂ cup balsamic vinegar   *¹/₂ teaspoon dried oregano*
4 garlic cloves, minced   *1 teaspoon salt*
1 teaspoon dried rosemary   *¹/₄ teaspoon black pepper*
1 teaspoon dried basil

1. Preheat the oven to 375°F.
2. Brush a baking sheet with the olive oil, wiping away any excess oil.
3. In a shallow bowl, combine the vinegar, garlic, herbs, salt, and pepper.
4. Slice the zucchini lengthwise into thick, 3- to 4-inch-long sticks.
5. Place the zucchini into the marinade and toss so that all the sticks are well coated. Arrange the zucchini on the baking sheet and roast for 25 minutes.

Spaghetti Squash
Serves 4 to 6

The stringy interior of spaghetti squash is a terrific substitute for flour-based pastas and is a good source of potassium, calcium, and vitamins A and C. It can be served with tomato sauce or tossed with oil and lemon as prepared here.

1 3- to 4-pound spaghetti squash
2 to 3 tablespoons olive oil
1 teaspoon lemon juice
1 tablespoon minced fresh basil
1 garlic clove, minced
Salt and black pepper

1. Preheat the oven to 350°F. Place the squash in a large baking pan with a little water in the bottom and bake for 25 minutes, or until a fork easily pierces the skin.
2. In a small bowl, combine the oil, lemon juice, basil, and garlic.
3. Cut the squash lengthwise and gently scoop out the seeds. Scoop out the strands of flesh from the center onto a platter and separate the strands with 2 forks. Toss lightly with the oil and lemon juice mixture. Add salt and pepper to taste and serve immediately. (It cools quickly.)

Stuffed Baked Potatoes
Serves 6

6 large potatoes (about 6
ounces each), baked
3 small garlic cloves, chopped
2 tablespoons chicken or
vegetable broth
1 cup nonfat milk, warmed
1½ cups nonfat ricotta cheese
1 teaspoon salt

½ teaspoon black pepper
½ teaspoon paprika
1 pound spinach, cleaned,
cooked, drained, and
chopped (2 10-ounce
packages frozen chopped
spinach, cooked and
drained, may also be used)

1. Preheat the oven to 350°F. Slice off the tops of the potatoes, scoop out the flesh, and transfer to a mixing bowl.
   Reserve the skins.
2. In a medium-sized saucepan, simmer the garlic in the
   broth until softened, about 3 minutes. In a large bowl,
   mash the potato with the milk, ricotta, sautéed garlic,
   salt, pepper, paprika, and spinach.
3. Stuff the potato mixture into the skins and place the
   skins in a shallow baking dish. Bake until heated
   through, about 20 minutes.

Roasted Vegetable Kabobs

Serves 4

Roasting is a marvelous technique for preparing succulent vegetables, and kabobs are a fun way of marrying flavors and textures. Experiment with vegetables such as broccoli or cauliflower florets, bell peppers, and various summer squashes and root vegetables.

2 teaspoons olive oil	8 cherry tomatoes
1 medium to large gold	8 pearl onions
zucchini, thickly sliced into	8 large mushroom caps
8 pieces	8 wooden shish kabob sticks

MARINADE

1/2 cup balsamic vinegar	1 teaspoon dried basil
4 garlic cloves, minced	1/2 teaspoon dried oregano
1 teaspoon dried rosemary	Salt and black pepper, to taste

1. Preheat the oven broiler to 450°F.
2. Brush a baking sheet with the olive oil.
3. Skewer the vegetables onto the kabob sticks, alternating the various vegetables.
4. In a small bowl, combine the vinegar, garlic, herbs, salt, and pepper.
5. Place the kabobs in the marinade and let sit for 20 minutes to an hour.
6. Roast the kabobs for 15 to 20 minutes, turning occasionally, or until the vegetables are tender but not mushy. Serve as hors d'oeuvres or with chicken or fish and a baked potato.

Low-Fat Artichokes
Serves 4

Artichokes are delicately flavored, low-calorie treats that don't need fats like butter, cheese, or oil. They can be eaten as snacks or as the vegetable portion of a meal, and are equally tasty hot or cold.

4 medium-sized artichokes	*$^1/_2$ cup lemon juice*
$^1/_4$ teaspoon black pepper	*3 cups chicken or vegetable*
4 garlic cloves, crushed	*broth*

1. Rinse the artichokes in a large bowl of cold water. Cut the stems off at the base.
2. In a small bowl, combine the pepper, garlic, and lemon juice and mix well.
3. Gently part the leaves of the artichokes and sprinkle the spiced lemon juice between them.
4. Place the chicken broth in a large pot. Add artichokes, base side down. Cover and simmer 30 minutes, or until the inner leaves pull out easily.
5. Serve with the broth or refrigerate and serve cold.

Stuffed Mushrooms
Serves 6 to 8

Stuffed mushrooms are a perennial favorite, but they are often stuffed with breadcrumbs and cheese. This version uses ground turkey and creative spicing to provide just the right mix of flavor and textures.

1 pound large mushrooms, stems removed and finely chopped

1 pound ground white turkey meat

4 teaspoons olive oil

3 garlic cloves, finely chopped

2 teaspoons finely chopped fresh basil

1 teaspoon white horseradish

1 teaspoon soy sauce

Black pepper to taste

1. Preheat the oven to 350°F. Brush or spray a cookie sheet with oil.
2. Combine the chopped mushroom stems and ground turkey and mix well.
3. Heat the oil in a skillet and briefly sauté the garlic. Add the turkey-mushroom mixture and cook over medium heat until the meat is thoroughly browned. Set the mixture aside to cool.
4. Combine the turkey-mushroom mixture with the basil, horseradish, soy sauce, and black pepper. Stuff the mushroom caps with the mixture.
5. Place the stuffed mushroom caps, stuffing side up, on the oiled cookie sheet. Bake for 18 minutes.

Green Beans with Sautéed Mushrooms
Serves 4

Mushrooms and green beans are a classic mix that goes well with almost any meal. For added crunch, sprinkle in some slivered almonds.

³/₄ pound green beans
1 tablespoon olive oil
2 small garlic cloves, chopped
2 teaspoons chopped fresh basil

¹/₄ teaspoon salt
Dash of Tabasco (optional)
1 cup sliced mushrooms
Dry white vermouth (optional)

1. Trim the ends off the beans and place in a steamer over about an inch of water. Cover and cook for 10 to 15 minutes, or until bright green and tender.
2. Heat the oil in a saucepan. Sauté the garlic, basil, salt, and Tabasco, if using, for a minute or two. Add the mushrooms and continue cooking, stirring occasionally, for 4 to 5 minutes, or until the mushrooms just begin to release their liquid. (If the mushrooms stick to the pan, you can add a dash of vermouth.)
3. Add the beans and mix well.

Grilled Vegetable Plate

Serves 4

Grilled vegetables can be served hot or cold, as an entrée or as a side dish. This recipe makes use of a Balsamic Vinaigrette and Spice Blend that have been made famous at the Chez Eddy restaurant in Houston, Texas.

1 medium zucchini, cut diagonally into ¼-inch slices

1 medium yellow squash, cut diagonally into ¼-inch slices

1 medium eggplant, cut crosswise into ¼-inch slices

1 medium red onion, cut into 8 wedges

4 plum tomatoes, halved lengthwise

8 small green onions, whole

1 large red bell pepper, cut into 8 wedges

2 teaspoons Spice Blend

½ cup Balsamic Vinaigrette

Nonstick cooking spray

SPICE BLEND

2 tablespoons chili powder

1 tablespoon black pepper

¼ teaspoon white pepper

1 tablespoon onion powder

1 tablespoon garlic powder

2 teaspoons ground cumin

1½ teaspoons fennel seed

1½ teaspoons mustard seed

⅛ teaspoon allspice

BALSAMIC
VINAIGRETTE

½ cup balsamic vinegar

½ teaspoon minced garlic

¾ teaspoon black pepper

1 tablespoon Dijon mustard

2 tablespoons olive oil

¾ cup nonfat yogurt

1. Spread the vegetables out in one layer on a tray or baking sheet.

2. Combine the Spice Blend ingredients in a blender.
3. Make the Balsamic Vinaigrette. In a small bowl, whisk together the vinegar, garlic, pepper, and mustard. Add the olive oil and yogurt, whisk together, and chill.
4. Brush the vegetables with the Balsamic Vinaigrette and sprinkle with the Spice Blend. Refrigerate 2 hours before grilling.
5. Apply another light coating of Balsamic Vinaigrette and grill, turning occasionally, until just tender. When ready to serve, alternate groups of vegetables on a dinner plate and drizzle each serving with 2 tablespoons Balsamic Vinaigrette.

Potato-Basil Crisp
Serves 4

Crispy without being fried, this variation on potato pancakes works just as well for breakfast (with a little fresh applesauce) as it does for dinner.

1 medium onion, finely chopped

4 cups shredded or grated peeled potatoes (about 6 medium)

2 tablespoons finely chopped fresh basil

½ teaspoon salt

Dash of white or black pepper

2 tablespoons canola or olive oil

1. In a large bowl, combine the onion, potatoes, basil, salt, and pepper. Mix well.
2. In a large skillet, warm 1 tablespoon oil. When the oil is hot, place half of the potato mixture in the skillet. Press down with a spatula to flatten and shape to the bottom. Cook about 15 minutes, or until the bottom is browned

evenly. Run a knife around the sides of the pan, then place a large plate over the pan. Using oven mitts, grip both sides of the pan with your hands and flip the crisp over onto the plate. Then gently slide the crisp's uncooked side onto the skillet. Cook 10 to 15 minutes more, then remove and repeat the procedure with the remaining potato mixture and oil.

Ratatouille
Serves 4 to 6

This rich vegetable stew can be served hot or cold. It makes a terrific side dish for lamb, beef, or fish, can be used as a stuffing for egg-white omelettes, and makes a complete meal when served over a baked potato or spaghetti squash. With a pot of ratatouille in your fridge, you'll never be at a loss for a quick, delicious, filling, and remarkably low-calorie meal.

1 medium eggplant
4 teaspoons olive oil
1 medium onion, sliced
3 garlic cloves, chopped
1 large green pepper, sliced
1 medium green or gold zucchini, sliced 1/4 inch thick
1/4 cup vegetable broth or dry white vermouth

3 tomatoes, peeled and chopped, or 1 28-ounce can whole peeled tomatoes in juice
2 teaspoons chopped fresh basil
1 teaspoon dried thyme
1 teaspoon dried oregano
Salt and pepper, to taste

1. Preheat the oven to 475°F.
2. Rinse the eggplant and slice in half lengthwise. Cut a long X in the skin of each half. Brush 2 teaspoons oil in a baking pan and place the eggplant, flat side down, in the pan. Bake for 10 to 15 minutes, or until the skin is

blistered and the eggplant is softened. Cool the eggplant, peel away the skin, and cut the halves into 1-inch cubes. Set aside. (Remember this step! It's the best way to prepare eggplant for use in other dishes as well, particularly eggplant parmigiana!)

3. Heat the remaining 2 teaspoons oil in a heavy pot. Add the onion and garlic and sauté until the onion is transparent, about 3 minutes. Add the pepper and cook 3 minutes more.

4. Add the eggplant and zucchini and mix the vegetables well. Add the broth and simmer for about 20 minutes, until the eggplant is tender and cooked through.

5. Add the tomatoes, herbs, and salt and pepper. Break apart the tomatoes with a spoon and simmer the mixture for 15 minutes. Taste and correct the seasoning as desired.

NOTE: If the ratatouille seems a bit watery, you can add a small can of tomato paste to thicken it. If it has a slightly bitter taste (which can sometimes happen with tomato dishes), grate a small carrot into the mix—it will counter the acidity of the tomato.

Steamed Asparagus with Sun-Dried Tomato Sauce

Serves 4

Asparagus is a delicate vegetable that is great when steamed or braised in vegetable stock. The addition of tart Sun-Dried Tomato Sauce makes this already delicious vegetable extraordinary.

SUN-DRIED TOMATO SAUCE

1¹/₄ cups chicken or vegetable broth	*1 tablespoon finely chopped fresh cilantro*
12 sun-dried tomatoes	*Black pepper*
1 tablespoon balsamic vinegar	*1 pound asparagus, washed*

1. In a small saucepan set over high heat, bring the broth to a boil. Add the tomatoes and set aside for 10 minutes, until the tomatoes rehydrate and become very soft.
2. Pour the tomatoes and broth into a blender and add the vinegar. Puree the mixture to form a thick, slightly chunky sauce.
3. Transfer the sauce to a bowl, stir in the cilantro, and season generously with pepper.
4. Break off the lower woody stems of the asparagus.
5. Place 2 cups of water in the bottom of a steamer, insert the steamer basket, and bring to a boil. When the steamer is filled with steam, add the asparagus, reduce the heat to medium, and steam until the asparagus are bright green and tender, 6 to 8 minutes. Transfer to a serving platter and top with the Sun-Dried Tomato Sauce.

SALADS

Salad Niçoise

Serves 4

Some versions of this dish call for anchovies, but this omits them, as well as half the oil in the dressing. The ingredients can be served tossed together in a salad bowl or arranged side by side on a platter.

2 medium red potatoes
1 head Boston or Bibb lettuce
1/4 pound French green beans
   (haricots verts)
8 cherry tomatoes, halved, or
   2 regular tomatoes,
   quartered

1 small green onion, chopped
1 hard-boiled egg, chopped
1/4 cup pitted black olives
1 6 1/2-ounce can white tuna,
   packed in water
1 teaspoon chopped parsley

DRESSING

1 garlic clove, minced
1/4 teaspoon dry mustard or
   1/2 teaspoon Dijon mustard
1/4 teaspoon dried tarragon

1/4 teaspoon dried dill
1/4 cup olive oil
3 tablespoons vegetable broth
   or water

1. Wash the potatoes well. Do not peel or slice.
2. Bring 2 inches of water to a boil in a medium pot and add the potatoes. Reduce the heat to medium and cook, covered, for 15 minutes. The potatoes should be tender when pierced with a fork. Quickly strain out the water and return the potatoes to the pan. Cover and let sit for 10 minutes. Remove the potatoes, quarter them, and chill.
3. Wash and dry the lettuce. Tear into large pieces.
4. Blanch the green beans by plunging them in boiling water for 1 minute, then chill.

5. Arrange all the salad ingredients in a bowl.
6. In a small bowl, combine the salad dressing ingredients. Drizzle the dressing over the assembled salad and toss thoroughly.

White Bean and Tuna Salad

Serves 4 to 6

Mixed salads like this one are a good way to work legumes into your diet while maintaining control over the amount of legumes you consume with each meal.

3 tablespoons olive oil
1 tablespoon Pommery
   mustard
$^1/_2$ teaspoon celery seed
$^1/_2$ teaspoon dried rosemary
2 garlic cloves, minced
2 6$^1/_2$-ounce cans tuna, packed
   in water

2 cups cooked white beans (or
   canned white beans, well
   rinsed)
$^1/_4$ teaspoon salt
$^1/_4$ teaspoon black pepper
Red leaf lettuce, for serving

1. In a large bowl, combine the oil, mustard, celery seed, rosemary, and garlic.
2. Drain the tuna. In a small bowl, mash the tuna with a fork to break it into small pieces. Add the tuna to the larger bowl and stir to mix.
3. Add the beans to the large bowl and lightly mix together. Add salt and pepper to taste.
4. Serve over a bed of red leaf lettuce.

SAUCES AND DRESSINGS

Herb Dressing for Greens

Makes 3 cups

This herb dressing works well over hot or cold green vegetables.

1 pound soft tofu
1½ cups water
2 tablespoons canola oil
2 tablespoons apple cider vinegar
2 tablespoons chopped dill

1 tablespoon dried mustard
1 tablespoon chopped basil
1 tablespoon chopped fresh mint
1 teaspoon dried thyme
Salt and pepper, to taste

In a blender or food processor, combine all the ingredients. Blend until smooth and well mixed. This can be refrigerated for up to 5 days.

White Bean and Roasted Garlic Sauce

This versatile sauce can be customized to fit almost any dish with the addition of just a few herbs. White beans are an excellent source of protein and soluble fiber (the type that has been shown to lower cholesterol), and they taste great, too.

4 to 6 garlic cloves, peeled
1 teaspoon olive oil
2 cups cooked white or navy beans (see Note)

¼ teaspoon salt or more, to taste
1 to 1½ cups chicken or vegetable broth

1. Preheat the oven to 350°F.
2. Brush the garlic cloves with oil and wrap in aluminum foil. Place in the oven and bake 20 minutes, or until the cloves are well softened.

3. Puree the beans, garlic, salt, and half of the broth, adding more broth as needed, until the mixture is creamy and smooth. Refrigerate.
4. When ready to serve, reheat the sauce, adding broth if necessary, over medium-low heat. Simmer for 5 minutes and serve.
5. When reheating for use, add additional herbs to the sauce as appropriate. For example, if you are going to use it on chicken, try adding basil and rosemary. For fish, add some fresh dill.

NOTE: If using canned beans, be sure to drain and rinse the beans thoroughly to wash off additives and any additional salt used in canning.

Low-Fat Tomato Sauce
Serves 4

This tomato sauce isn't just for pasta. Try it over fish, chicken cutlets, or even lightly sautéed vegetables. For a slightly heartier sauce, add some chopped green or red peppers and some sliced mushrooms along with the spices.

1 tablespoon olive oil	*$^1/_2$ teaspoon dried thyme*
1 small onion, finely diced	*Dry white vermouth or red*
2 garlic cloves, minced	*wine (optional)*
1 whole bay leaf	*1 28-ounce can whole*
2 teaspoons dried basil	*tomatoes in juice*
1 teaspoon chopped parsley	*Salt and pepper, to taste*

1. Heat the oil in a medium saucepan over low heat. Swirl it around so the bottom is coated with oil and then wipe up the excess with a paper towel. Add the onion and cook over medium heat until golden, about 5 minutes.
2. Add the garlic and cook 2 minutes.

3. Add the bay leaf, basil, parsley, and thyme. Cook 2 minutes. If the herbs are sticking to the pan, you can add just a splash of dry white vermouth or red wine.
4. Add the tomatoes and their juice. As they simmer, break the tomatoes into pieces with a spoon. Add the salt and pepper. Reduce the heat to low and let simmer partially covered for 20 minutes. Remove the bay leaf, taste, and adjust the seasoning as desired.

DESSERTS

Banana Cream
Serves 4

Banana Cream satisfies the need for something cool and creamy while providing much-needed potassium. You can customize this recipe by adding a frozen fresh peach or 1/4 cup frozen berries.

6 very ripe bananas
3 tablespoons cold water or orange juice

1/2 cup chopped walnuts, pecans, or almonds

1. Peel the bananas and freeze. (They can be left overnight, or put them in the freezer in the morning to prepare in the evening.)
2. Put the frozen bananas in a food processor or blender and quickly puree, adding water or juice 1 tablespoon at a time until the bananas are the consistency of ice cream. Divide into 4 portions, sprinkle with nuts, and serve immediately.

Poached Apples and Pears with Berry Sauce
Serves 4
This recipe is a nice way of making your daily fruit serving into an elegant and delicious dessert. It will also work without the berries during times of the year when berries are not in season.

4 cups apple or apple-
   raspberry juice
1 cup finely chopped
   strawberries or raspberries
2 lemon slices

1 1-inch cinnamon stick
$1/2$ teaspoon vanilla extract
2 whole golden or red
   Delicious apples, peeled
2 whole Bosc pears, peeled

1. In a medium saucepan, combine the apple juice, berries, lemon slices, cinnamon stick, and vanilla extract. Bring to a boil over high heat, then reduce to a simmer. Add the apples and pears, cover, and cook 12 minutes. The fruit is done when a fork slides easily into the flesh. Remove the fruit with a slotted spoon and set aside in a covered dish to keep warm, or bring to room temperature and chill.
2. Continue cooking the juice and berries until the liquid is reduced to a thick sauce, about 25 minutes. Divide the fruit among 4 plates and drizzle the sauce over each serving.

Fresh Fruit Compote

Makes 4 cups

This fiber-rich compote is a good homemade substitute for commercial all-fruit preserves, and can be served over waffles, hot cereal, muffins, or by itself as a dessert.

4 cups apple juice or apple
   juice combination
2 golden or red Delicious
   apples, cored and coarsely
   chopped
1 Bosc pear, cored and
   coarsely chopped
1 peach or 2 fresh apricots,
   pitted and coarsely chopped

1 fresh fig (or 4 dried
   unsulphured figs), coarsely
   chopped
$^1/_2$ cup seasonal berries
$^1/_4$ cup raisins
$^1/_2$ teaspoon cinnamon

1. Place all the ingredients in a medium pot and bring to a boil over medium heat.
2. Reduce the heat to a simmer and cook until the fruit is very thick and syrupy, about 30 minutes. Refrigerate.

Fresh Fruit Pie with Nut Crust
Serves 8
This is a delicious, no-cook alternative to pies with fatty flour-based crusts. The crunchy nut crust is a good source of protein, and the sweet fresh fruit filling is rich in antioxidant vitamins.

CRUST

1 cup almonds

1 cup walnuts

$^1/_3$ cup raisins

$^1/_4$ cup apple juice

FILLING

2 bananas

1 tablespoon freshly squeezed lemon juice

2 to 3 kiwifruits, peeled and sliced

1 quart fresh strawberries, sliced

1. Place the nuts and raisins in a blender or food processor and pulse until they are chopped well but not too fine (they should resemble pebbles, not flour). Add the apple juice and pulse on and off for a few seconds. Pour the nut mixture into a glass pie plate and press out to shape a crust.
2. Slice the bananas and spread them inside the bottom of the nut crust, pressing slightly. Sprinkle with the lemon juice to prevent the bananas from turning brown. Layer the kiwifruits on top of the bananas, pressing slightly. Repeat with the strawberries.
3. Chill for at least 1 hour. Carefully slice and serve.

Fruit Smoothies
Serves 1

Fruit smoothies are a nutritious way of satisfying your ice cream cravings and getting your needed allotment of fruit. They can be made with just about any fruit and are a wonderful quick dessert on hot summer nights. For added calcium and protein, add ¼ cup plain or flavored low-fat yogurt.

The basic instructions for building a smoothie are simple: Crush about ½ cup of ice (about 6 cubes) in a blender, then add the other ingredients and blend until smooth.

PEACH SMOOTHIE

2 peaches, peeled and pitted
1 banana

¼ teaspoon vanilla extract
Dash of ground nutmeg

BERRY SMOOTHIE

½ cup blueberries,
  raspberries, blackberries,
  or sliced strawberries
1 banana

¼ cup apple juice
¼ teaspoon maple syrup
  (optional)

MUFFINS

Note: These recipes are only for those who do not have a problem with baked goods.

The Mayor's Muffins

Makes about 15 muffins

These fiber-rich muffins get their sweetness from nutrient-rich bananas and molasses. A single muffin, along with a piece of fresh fruit and some juice, makes a quick, filling breakfast on even the most rushed of mornings.

1 cup Fiber One cereal
1 cup all-purpose whole wheat flour
1 teaspoon baking soda
2/3 cup raisins
1 egg
1/2 teaspoon cinnamon

1/4 cup molasses
3 to 4 bananas, mashed (about 1 1/2 cups)
3/4 cup nonfat cottage cheese
1 tablespoon margarine (preferably made with safflower or canola oil)

1. Preheat the oven to 350°F.
2. In a large bowl, combine the cereal, flour, and baking soda and mix well.
3. Add the raisins to the flour mixture and combine thoroughly.
4. In a large bowl, whip the egg until frothy. Add the cinnamon and molasses and whip.
5. Puree the bananas and cottage cheese in a blender or food processor if possible and add to the egg mixture. Stir until the mixture is smooth.
6. Gradually stir in the flour mixture.
7. Pour the batter into lightly greased (or nonstick) muffin tins. Bake for 1 hour, or until the muffins are springy to the touch. Let cool in the tins for 5 minutes, then turn out onto a rack.

Complementary Light and Airy Muffins
Makes 8 muffins

These fluffy muffins are a bit like popovers. They are low enough in carbohydrates to prevent cravings in those who are carbohydrate sensitive, but tasty and filling enough to satisfy the need for an occasional bread product.

1/2 tablespoon canola oil
4 eggs, separated
1/2 teaspoon cream of tartar
1/4 cup low-fat cottage cheese

2 tablespoons soy flour
1 packet artificial sweetener
*   (aspartame or saccharin)*

1. Preheat the oven to 300°F. Brush the muffin cups with the oil.
2. Beat the egg whites with an electric mixer until frothy. Add the cream of tartar and continue beating until stiff peaks form.
3. Combine the egg yolks, cottage cheese, soy flour, and sweetener. Fold the mixture carefully into the egg whites.
4. Fill each muffin cup 2/3 full of batter. Bake the muffins for about 30 minutes, until they are golden brown and spring back when touched with a finger.

RECIPE SOURCES

Grateful acknowledgment is made to the following individuals and publishers for permission to reprint their recipes.

- Jacki Deena Tutelman
  Roasted Vegetable Kabobs, Scallops with White Wine and Lemon.
- Catherine Heusel
  Low-Fat Artichokes, One-Pot Chicken and Stock.
- Bea Radomsky
  Vegetable Lasagna.
- Susan Knightly
  Simple Vegetable Stock, Ratatouille, No-Fat "Fried" Zucchini Sticks, Salad Niçoise, Low-Fat Tomato Sauce, White Bean and Roasted Garlic Sauce.
- *The Carbohydrate Addict's Diet* by Rachael F. Heller, Ph.D., and Richard F. Heller, Ph.D. (New York: Signet Books, 1993)
  Green Beans with Sautéed Mushrooms, Stuffed Mushrooms, Herbed Turkey Burgers, Complementary Light and Airy Muffins.
- *Cooking for a New Earth* by Carl Jerome (New York: Henry Holt and Company, 1993)
  Steamed Asparagus with Sun-Dried Tomato Sauce
- *Eat More, Weigh Less* by Dean Ornish, M.D. (New York: HarperCollins, 1993)
  Stuffed Baked Potatoes.

- *Food for Recovery* by Joseph D. Beasley, M.D., and Susan Knightly (New York: Crown Publishers, 1993)
  Potato-Basil Crisp, Spaghetti Squash, White Bean and Tuna Salad, Broccoli Soup, Blender Gazpacho, Herbed Chicken Breasts, Grilled Chicken Salad, Herb Dressing for Greens, Poached Apples and Pears with Berry Sauce, Fresh Fruit Pie with Nut Crust, Banana Cream, Fresh Fruit Compote, Poached Fish with Vegetables, Baked Salmon Steaks, Garlic Shrimp.
- *The Living Heart Cookbook* by Antonio M. Gotto, M.D., Helen Roe, and the staff of the Chez Eddy Restaurant (New York: Fireside Books, 1991)
  Grilled Vegetable Plate.
- *Moosewood Restaurant Cooks at Home* by The Moosewood Collective (New York: Fireside Books, 1994)
  Braised Fish with Artichoke Hearts and Red Peppers.

THIN TASTES BETTER
RECOMMENDED BRANDS

Winners of the Thin Tastes Better Awards for America's Best Diet Foods

Over the last decade, many companies have developed healthy alternatives to the high-fat, high-sugar, high-calorie foods that line supermarket shelves. The following brands are among my clients' favorites, and are widely available nationally. Winners of the *Thin Tastes Better* Awards are marked with an asterisk. Many supermarkets' "house brands" now include reasonably priced low-fat, low-calorie foods as well.

FOOD TYPE	WHAT TO LOOK FOR	BRAND NAME
BREAKFAST FOODS		
Cereals (cold)	whole grain	Kellogg's Special K
	no added sugar	Healthy Choice
	no fat	Multi-Grain Flakes
		Kellogg's Product 19
		Post Grape-Nuts
		Cheerios
Cereals (hot)	whole grain	H-O Instant Oatmeals
	no added sugar	*Instant Quaker
	low salt	Oatmeal
	no fat	*Pritikin Hearty hot
		cereal

FOOD TYPE	WHAT TO LOOK FOR	BRAND NAME
Pancake Syrups		Aunt Jemima Light reduced-calorie syrup product
Waffles	no fat whole grain no added sugar	*Aunt Jemima Lite Waffles *Kellog's Eggo Special K fat-free waffles
LUNCH/ DINNER FOODS		
Sandwich Breads	whole grain high protein high fiber less than 40 calories a slice	any brand
Cheeses	no fat no cholesterol less than 30 calories a slice	Borden Lite Line (all varieties) Weight Watchers Fat Free (all varieties) *Smart Beat (all varieties) *Alpine Lace (all varieties) Borden Fat Free (all varieties) Kraft Free Singles *Healthy Choice Fat Free

FOOD TYPE	WHAT TO LOOK FOR	BRAND NAME
Cheeses (cont.)		Laughing Cow Light Mini Babybel
		Polly-O Free Natural Nonfat Mozzarella Cheese
		Polly-O Free Natural Nonfat Ricotta Cheese
		ANY nonfat cottage cheese
		Swiss Knight Lite
Cold Cuts	no fat less than 30 calories a slice	Healthy Choice Low Fat Deli Thin Sliced
		*Healthy Choice frankfurters
		*Hillshire Farms Deli Select
		Oscar Mayer Light cold cuts
		Hormel Light frankfurters
Apple Sauce		*Mott's Natural Style
Poultry		*Swanson Whole Chicken in water
Frozen Foods	low or no fat low salt less than 350 calories for men, less than 250 calories for women	*Healthy Choice frozen dinners
		Weight Watchers Smart Ones
		Lean Cuisine frozen dinners

FOOD TYPE	WHAT TO LOOK FOR	BRAND NAME
Frozen Foods (cont.)		Lean Cuisine Lunch Express
		Stouffer's Right Course
		Weight Watchers Ultimate 200
		Gorton's Select (prespiced fish fillets)
		*Green Giant frozen vegetable patties
Pastas	whole grain	Contadina High Protein
		De Bole's Natural Gourmet
		Pritikin whole wheat spaghetti
Soups	low or no fat	*Health Valley Fat-Free Soups
	low salt	Progresso Healthy Classics
	additive free	Campbell's Healthy Request
		Herb-Ox Very Low Sodium Instant Broth and Seasonings
		Lipton's Cup-A-Soup (50-calorie variety)

FOOD TYPE	WHAT TO LOOK FOR	BRAND NAME
Soups (cont.)		Ultra Slim Fast instant soups
		MBT instant broths (low sodium)
Cooking Oils	cold-pressed	*Pam olive oil spray
	extra virgin	*Pam butter spray
	first press	Hain
		Loriva
		Spectrum Naturals
		Weight Watchers Cooking Spray (canola oil)
Margarines		*Smart Beat
Flavorings		*Butter Buds
Fruit Butters	no added sugar	Eden Farms
	sweetened with fruit juice	Walnut Acres
	no corn syrup	
Fruit Toppings	no added sugar	Polaner All Fruit
		Walnut Acres
		Berry Best Farms
		Cascadian Farms
		R. W. Knudsen
		Sorrell Ridge
Mayonnaise	low/no fat	*Kraft Free nonfat mayonnaise dressing
		Smart Beat nonfat mayonnaise dressing

FOOD TYPE	WHAT TO LOOK FOR	BRAND NAME
Mayonnaise (cont.)		Weight Watchers Light Mayonnaise
Mustard		Hellman's Dijonnaise Creamy Mustard Blend
Salad Dressings	low/no fat no added sugar less than 70 calories per 2-tablespoon serving	Kraft Fat-Free dressings *Weight Watchers Salad Celebrations in packets Smart Temptations Healthy Sensation! Wishbone Lite Italian Dressing *Jardine's fat-free dressings
Salsas	no added sugar no fat no corn syrup	Cowboy Caviar *Jardine's fat-free salsas
Sauces (spaghetti)	no added sugar no corn syrup low salt no fat	*Healthy Choice pasta sauce Ci'Bella Eden (organic only) Enrico Pritikin Tree of Life
Crackers		*Jardine's fat-free crackers
SNACKS/DESSERTS		
Gelatins	no sugar	JELL-O Sugar Free

FOOD TYPE	WHAT TO LOOK FOR	BRAND NAME
Gelatins (cont.)		Estee low-calorie gelatins
		Featherweight Sweet Pretenders
Hot chocolate	no sugar	Weight Watchers Hot Cocoa
		Swiss Miss Diet Hot Cocoa
		Carnation diet hot chocolate
Chocolate Shakes	no sugar	*Alba Reduced Calorie Dairy Shake Mix
	low/no fat	Weight Watchers Chocolate Fudge Shake Mix
Chocolate Syrups	no fat	Wax Orchards
	low/no sugar	Canyon Ranch
Popcorn		*Nude Food No Fat popcorn (Robert's American Gourmet)
		Weight Watchers butter-flavored popcorn (individual size servings)
Frozen Desserts	no added sugar	Weight Watchers Chocolate Treat
	no/low fat	*Chocolate Mousse low-fat
	less than 70 calories a serving	

FOOD TYPE	WHAT TO LOOK FOR	BRAND NAME
Frozen Desserts (cont.)		chocolate flavored ice cream
		*Berries & Cream Mousse low-fat ice cream
		Popsicle sugar-free fruit ice pops
		*Fiberry berry snack bar (Interior Design)
		FrozFruit any berry flavor lemon lime
		*Crystal Light Pops
		Dole No Sugar Added Fruit Juice Quiescently Frozen Juice Bars
		Welch's Fruit Juice Bars
		*Häagen Dazs Frozen Yogurt Bar (90–100 calories)
BEVERAGES		
Drinks	no sugar	*Diet Rite sodas (the best diet sodas in America)
Drink Mixes		
Sodas		*Crystal Light

FOOD TYPE	WHAT TO LOOK FOR	BRAND NAME
Drinks		*RC diet cola
Drink Mixes		Diet Orangina
Sodas (cont.)		Schweppes diet raspberry ginger ale
		*Arizona Diet Iced Tea (the best diet tea in America)
		Lipton's sugar-free iced tea
		*Jeff's Diet Chocolate Egg Creams
Supplements	(always check with your physician about vitamins and food supplements)	I use the following:
		*Interior Design vitamin line
		*Prime 1 Herbal Food Supplement (Prime Quest Int'l, Monterey, CA)

NUTRITIONISTS, WEIGHT-LOSS CENTERS, AND SPAS

You, like many men and women, may feel that you just can't do it when it comes to weight control. That's not at all the case. For you, it may simply be that you can't do it *alone.* So I would encourage you to seek out a weight program or health professional. You can check with your local hospital to see if it has a weight program on-site. Or you can go to a commercial weight-loss program, whether it be Weight Watchers, Diet Center, Jenny Craig, or any other reputable service. Keep in mind, however, that these programs must meet the needs of a large, diverse population. But it will not be difficult to reshape the program for your own needs, using *Thin Tastes Better.*

For highly personal attention, you may want to consider seeing a nutritionist. Some may even come to your home to help you rearrange the food in your refrigerator and evaluate the foods you keep on your shelves.

Be aware, however, that since most states do not require nutritionists to be licensed or certified, you could fall prey to some fly-by-night entrepreneur with a mail-order degree. The solution: Make sure the nutritionist you see is a registered dietitian (RD), preferably with a bachelor's degree in nutrition or dietetics from an accredited college or university. A good place to start: the American Dietetic Association's Nutrition Hotline, at (800) 366-1655, staffed by RDs who answer questions and offer food-smart advice on everything from snacking to food allergies to nutrition for fitness. They also provide names of nutritionists in your area.

One caveat: Some RDs will probably give you the party line about eating lots of pasta, breads, and other grains and starches or following the USDA Food Pyramid. You must choose your nutritionist carefully, keeping in mind you want someone who will respect your body's unique needs and help you stick to the lessons learned in your Eating Print. When it comes to the war against fat, nutritionists, dietitians, and your physician are all out on the front lines, and they can be of great assistance in your efforts to control your weight. Do not hesitate to use their services.

If you think you need some serious in-house supervision, you might want to consider attending a residential program at a weight-loss center. Weight-loss clinics serve those who need to lose from just a few stubborn pounds to a couple hundred, providing their guests with nutrition information, behavior modification techniques, and exercise routines. While some guests may have received such advice and information before, sometimes the simple act of getting away from the usual day-to-day stresses in their lives is what does the trick and they take the health advice to heart like never before.

Perhaps getting away from it all will work to jump-start your return to thin. Don't dismiss this option completely out of hand because you think that all such clinics are only for the rich and famous. True, many can be pricey, but your insurance may cover fees for medical services like exams and tests; the remainder of your expenses may be covered, too, if your doctor considers your weight a serious health risk. Check your policy.

Excellent weight-loss centers, often recommended by health professionals, include the following.

- Duke University Diet and Fitness Center, 804 West Trinity Avenue, Durham, NC 27701; (800) 362-8446; fax (919) 684-6176. One of my personal favorites, the Duke facility is headed by Dr. Michael Hamilton, an exceptionally gifted and caring physician, who heads a talented staff.
- Green Mountain at Fox Run, Box 164, Fox Lane, Ludlow, VT 05149; (800) 448-8106 or (802) 228-8885.
- The Hilton Head Health Institute, 14 Valencia Road, Box 7138, Hilton Head Island, SC 29938-7138; (800) 292-2440 or (803) 785-7292.
- Pritikin Longevity Centers, 1910 Ocean Front Walk, Santa Monica, CA 90405; (800) 421-9911 or (310) 450-5433. Also at 5875 Collins Avenue, Miami Beach, FL 33140; (800) 327-4914 or (305) 865-8645.
- Structure House, 3017 Pickett Road, Durham, NC 27705; (800) 553-0052 or (919) 688-7379.

Spas can also be a great chance to get away from it all and get in touch with your physical and nutritional needs. All of us sometimes need to step out of our normal day-to-day life, with its pressures and food obsessions, and into a protective environment where we can recharge our energies and refocus our attention on caring for our bodies and ourselves in a loving way. I urge anyone who is having trouble sticking to a weight program to take a long weekend, or a week, if possible, in such an environment. It can do wonders for your control.

Again, not all spa cuisine or advice may be in sync with your Eating Print, so follow what you know about your control. Such places can be especially useful if you have lost control with a particular type of food (e.g., sweets) and need to discover that you can, in fact, live without it one day at a time. Gradually, you'll see the craving start to disappear. Thus renewed, you can return to normal life stronger and better able to deal with that food.

One of the best spas, in my opinion, is Canyon Ranch, 8600 East Rockcliff Road, Tucson, AZ 85715; (800) 742-9000 or (602) 749-9000. Also at 165 Kemble Street, Lenox, MA 01240; (800) 326-7080 or (413) 637-4100. This health and fitness resort has a number of programs that each emphasize different fitness and nutritional concerns; the food served, by and large, follows the white and green watchwords of the Food Control Eating Plan. I especially like their Life Enhancement Program. I have worked on numerous occasions with the staff of Canyon Ranch's Berkshire campus in Massachusetts and I have found the medical director, Dr. Stephanie Beling, and their programs to be topnotch and most helpful.

Another good choice is The Greenhouse, Box 1144, Arlington, TX 76004; (817) 640-4000. Or inquire about La Costa Resort and Spa, 2100 Costa del Mar Road, Carlsbad, CA 92009; (800) 854-5000 or (619) 438-9111.

If you're interested in finding out more about spas in a certain region of the country, check out the following books: *The Best Spas* by Theodore B. Van Itallie, M.D., and Leila Hadley (New York: Perennial, 1988) and *The Ultimate Spa Book* by Pam Martin Sarnoff (New York: Warner Books, 1989).

FOR MORE INFORMATION

COOKBOOKS
Cookbooks have changed a lot in the last ten years. Rich, fatty recipes are rapidly being replaced by light, flavorful dishes. New cookbooks appear on the shelves almost daily, but these are among the best I've found; some of their recipes are featured beginning on page 255.

- Beasley, Joseph D., M.D., and Susan Knightly. *Food For Recovery.* New York: Crown Publishers, 1993.
- Brody, Jane. *Jane Brody's Good Food Book.* New York: Bantam, 1987.
- Daley, Rosie. *In the Kitchen with Rosie.* New York: Knopf, 1994.
- Gotto, Antonio M., M.D., Helen Roe, and the staff of the Chez Eddy Restaurant. *The Living Heart Cookbook.* New York: Fireside Books, 1991.
- Heller, Rachael F., Ph.D., and Richard F. Heller, Ph.D. *The Carbohydrate Addict's Diet.* New York: Signet Books, 1993.
- Jerome, Carl. *Cooking for a New Earth.* New York: Henry Holt and Company, 1993.
- The Moosewood Collective. *Moosewood Restaurant Cooks at Home.* New York: Fireside Books, 1994.
- Ornish, Dean, M.D. *Eat More, Weigh Less.* New York: HarperCollins, 1993.

FITNESS

Health magazines provide a wealth of fitness and health information, including precise how-tos each month for exercises and fitness programs. Whether you are male, female, a novice, or an experienced athlete, you're bound to find a magazine tailored to your needs at a newsstand near you. Some of the best for women include *Self, Shape,* and *Fitness.* (There's also good overall health coverage in *Allure* and *New Woman.*) Men, check out *Men's Health* and *Men's Fitness.* And for both men and women, *Longevity, Runner's World,* and *Walking.* Or look for these books.

- Cooper, Kenneth H., M.D., M.P.H. *Running Without Fear: How to Reduce the Risk of Heart Attack and Sudden Death During Aerobic Exercise.* New York: M. Evans & Co., 1985.
- Eliot, Robert S., M.D., and Dennis L. Breo. *Is It Worth Dying For? A Self-Assessment Program to Make Stress Work For You and Not Against You.* Toronto: Bantam Books, 1984.
- Lebow, Fred, Gloria Averbuch, and friends. *The New York Road Runners Club Complete Book of Running.* New York: Random House, 1994.
- Rippe, James M., M.D., with Patricia Amend. *The Exercise Exchange Program.* New York: Simon and Schuster, 1992.
- Rippe, James M., M.D., and Carol A. Ward. *The Rockport Walking Program.* New York: Prentice Hall, 1989.
- Wilmore, Jack H., Ph.D. *Sensible Fitness.* Champaign, IL: Leisure Press, 1986.

FOOD

- Gittleman, Ann Louise. *Guess What Came to Dinner: Parasites and Your Health.* Garden City Park, NY: Avery Publishing Group, 1993.
- Jacobson, Michael F., Ph.D., and Sarah Fritschner. *The Fast-Food Guide: What's Good, What's Bad and How to Tell the Difference.* New York: Workman Publishing, 1986.
- Winter, Ruth, M.S. *A Consumer's Dictionary of Food Additives.* New York: Crown Publishers, 1989.

HEALTH

Cutting-edge research and the latest developments in health and nutrition are reported in two excellent newsletters: *Nutrition Action Healthletter* from the Center for Science in the Public Interest, (202) 332-9110, and the *Tufts University Diet & Nutrition Letter,* (800) 274-7581.

- Cooper, Kenneth H., M.D. *Dr. Kenneth H. Cooper's Antioxidant Revolution.* Nashville: Thomas Nelson Publishers, 1994.
- Kembel, Julie Waltz. *Winning the Weight and Wellness Game.* Tucson, AZ: Northwest Learning Associates, Inc., 1993.
- Klein, Arthur C., and Dava Sobel. *Backache Relief: The Ultimate Second Opinion from Back-Pain Sufferers Nationwide Who Share Their Successful Healing Experiences.* New York: Signet, 1985.
- Logue, A. W. *The Psychology of Eating and Drinking.* New York: W. H. Freeman & Company, 1986.
- Nagler, Willibald, M.D., and Irene von Estorff, M.D. *Dr. Nagler's Body Maintenance and Repair Book.* New York: Simon and Schuster, 1987.

- Root, Leon, M.D. *No More Aching Back.* New York: Villard Books, 1990.
- Sacker, Ira M., M.D., and Marc A. Zimmer, Ph.D. *Dying to Be Thin: Understanding and Defeating Anorexia Nervosa and Bulimia—A Practical, Lifesaving Guide.* New York: Warner Books, 1987.
- Sarno, John E., M.D. *Healing Back Pain: The Mind-Body Connection.* New York: Warner Books, 1991.
- Simopoulos, Artemis P., M.D., Victor Herbert, M.D., J.D., and Beverly Jacobson. *Genetic Nutrition: Designing a Diet Based on Your Family Medical History.* New York: Macmillan Publishing Company, 1993.
- Waterhouse, Debra, M.P.H., R.D. *Outsmarting the Female Fat Cell.* New York: Hyperion, 1993.

MEDITATION AND YOGA

- Benson, Herbert G., M.D., and Miriam Z. Klipper. *The Relaxation Response.* New York: Avon, 1976.
- Kabat-Zinn, Jon. *Wherever You Go, There You Are: Mindfulness Meditation in Everyday Life.* New York: Hyperion, 1994.
- *Molly Fox's Yoga* (series of videos offering a variety of nonimpact workouts), Parade Video. Available in most video stores.
- Ornish, Dean, M.D. *Eat More, Weigh Less.* New York: HarperCollins, 1993.
- *Total Beauty and Fitness* (video featuring Raquel Welch, who teaches twenty-eight intermediate to advanced postures), HBO Video. Available in most video stores.
- *Yoga Companion* (video from Yoga Journal Book & Tape Source, 2054 University Ave., Berkeley, CA 94704-1082; 800-359-YOGA).

- *Yoga Journal's Yoga for Beginners* (video and introductory booklet available at Yoga Journal Book & Tape Source, Berkeley, CA).

WEIGHT, FOOD, AND CULTURE
- Stacey, Michelle. *Consumed: Why Americans Love, Hate, and Fear Food.* New York: Simon and Schuster, 1994.
- Visser, Margaret. *The Rituals of Dinner: The Origins, Evolution, Eccentricities and Meaning of Table Manners.* New York: Penguin Books, 1991.
- Wolf, Naomi. *The Beauty Myth: How Images of Beauty Are Used Against Women.* New York: Anchor Books, 1992.